Breaking the Pattern

Breaking
the Pattern

The 5 Principles You
Need to Remodel Your Life

Charles Stuart Platkin

Red Mill Press

New York City

Published by
Red Mill Press
Old Chelsea Station
PO Box 1272
New York, New York 10113

Library of Congress Cataloging-in-Publication Data

Platkin, Charles S.

ISBN 0-9711503-0-3

1. Self Improvement   2. Change (Psychology)   3. Weight Loss

Printed in the United States of America

Cover Design by Blue Design
Design Consultant Benjy Kile

Acknowledgements

There are many people who have given their support during the writing of this book. No one writes a book alone and there are many people whom I wish to thank for their contribution, support, and dedication.

I primarily thank Meredith Abreu for her being an amazing critic, editor, and "test dummy" for the book, as well as for her belief in me—through thick and thin.

I thank Connie deSwaan for her patience—her phenomenal editorial capabilities and her insistence that the writing truly reflect my thoughts.

I thank Janet Allon for helping get this book into a believable format, and Brian Frank and Victoria Blake for taking the time to sit at my kitchen table and gather and sort through thousands of pages of research.

This book is dedicated to my parents,
who provided me with great role models;
to my friend and mentor Carole McCarthy;
and finally to the person who allowed me to
reflect my true self, my soul mate, Shannon.

Contents

Chapter Six

ACHIEVEMENT

Chapter Seven

Chapter Eight

Introduction

What One Can Imagine, One Can Achieve.

It's hard to pinpoint the exact genesis of this book.

In a way, it begins with my life as a thinking adult responsible for making my way in the world. Even though I had some success, I couldn't help but wonder if there were a road map or instruction manual to living right—an infallible guide that would tell me what to do, how to act, and what to avoid. Of course, there was none.

I'd been in several romantic relationships that were not successful. Each relationship seemed to end the same way; the personalities of the women shared a common theme—and, of course, I blamed them for what went wrong. In addition, I had been fat most of my life. In my 30s, I was nearly 50 pounds overweight. I tried every diet known, but they were all no good— and I blamed the diets. Professionally, I had been involved in several entrepreneurial partnerships. Each partnership ended badly, and all had a common theme. Again, I thought it was all of them that were at fault. I took no responsibility for the fact that I had chosen these women, these diets, and these business partners. It was much easier to make excuses, or to blame others or destiny for my lot in life. In a more concrete way, the idea for this book started as a letter I wrote to a friend I hadn't seen in the 14 years since our graduation from college.

It seemed like a simple task to write Marie—just a newsy missive about what I'd been up to since we last saw each other. I envisioned only a few pages. Once I began writing, the simple task grew into a monumental undertaking. If you've lived into your 30s and beyond, you understand how this can happen—in telling the news, you become deeply autobiographical and reveal more about yourself than you'd expected. At 35 years old, I was ripe for self-reflection and my friend was getting every image of me.

This letter to my friend helped me to see the story of my life a little more clearly. Writing it helped me synthesize and clarify certain issues and thoughts that had long interested me, or *patterns of behavior.* In fact, I'd already put in years of research on certain patterns, such as the effects of an exaggerated fear of failure, how one does or doesn't take responsibility for one's own life, how step-by-step goal—planning works for optimum performance, and the results of various strategies for living a life of achievement. I was very focused on ways to improve my life.

I was trying to figure out how these ideas impact each other and how they could be combined and harnessed positively to bring about greater satisfaction—in my own life and in the lives of others. It became clear that to make meaningful changes in my own life, I had to find a way to consciously bring these patterns to the surface for closer examination. To change, I knew I had to not only go wide, but also go very deep.

After years of research, self-reflection, self-examination, and my share of failures, I realized that many of the things occurring in my life were beginning to look familiar. I found something they had in common, that is, patterns and outcomes I had experienced before, which drove me to the same places that I didn't want to see again. *They were repeats.* It felt as if I were having that vaguely annoying realization that I've already seen the film I just rented, remembered that I disliked it the first time, and definitely didn't want to sit through it again.

Of course, I am not the only one repeating patterns like these. I wanted to know how others dealt with their own patterns and therefore I started asking questions. Through interviews and discussions with professionals and friends, from reading about the lives of people who had struggled to succeed, and by being an interested observer, I've learned that *most of us repeat and maintain certain patterns throughout our lives, and that we often do so unconsciously.* The experiences that patterns produce may seem different and unrelated, but if you look at the effects, you'll see this sense of difference is an illusion. The experiences may have different casts of characters, are changed by different times and places in slightly altered circumstances, but if you are still trapped by patterns that don't serve you well, it's all the same.

We've all been there, and have told ourselves time and time again:

▸ "It's that lousy diet—I knew it wasn't going to help me lose weight."
▸ "I don't understand it. I always get the worst bosses. I'm so unlucky."
▸ "This is my fourth relationship in four years. Aren't there any good men out there?"

These observations of behavior, others'—and my own—led me to an inescapable conclusion, which formed the basis of this book:

When we examine our successes and failures honestly and carefully, we can see the outline of very distinct patterns. By being aware of these patterns, we can analyze them, break them down, and focus on not repeating the negative behavior that has led us to failure and disappointment. We can also learn to capitalize on our positive patterns, thereby making huge advances in both our personal and professional lives.

I have found it impossible to break a behavioral pattern by simply wishing or willing it so. For long-term change, the only way to "break the pattern" is by following the five critical Principles required for real change—and for changing the way you live. The following are the five Principles to help you change and remodel your life:

1. *Patterns.* Here you will review and evaluate various stages of your life, reflect on those stages and, especially, look for your underlying negative patterns.
2. *Failure.* To be successful you can't be afraid to risk failure. Failure is an opportunity to learn and grow, and is an integral part of achievement, not separate from it.
3. *Responsibility.* By focusing on individual responsibility, you can learn to accept the fact that you are responsible for the choices you make in your life. This opens you up to opportunity—only then is real change possible.
4. *Goals.* Reaching your goals requires planning ahead and developing a strategy. When you set goals and believe in them, you have a greater likelihood of achieving them. Your goals must also be S.M.A.R.T.—Specific, Motivating, Achievable, Rewarding, and Tactical. Achievement is not something that happens to anyone by accident—it is planned for, visualized and relentlessly pursued.
5. *Achievement.* Understanding that achievement is the result of action-oriented behavior will encourage you to develop tactics and strategies such as being proactive, learning personal values, paradigm shifting, and being "opportunity ready."

These Principles are the components that have helped me overcome my negative patterns and live a happier and more rewarding life. This book offers concrete techniques to help you evaluate and assess your behavior and actions so that you can make a difference in your life.

One underlying question these Principles will answer is: *Why do certain people achieve their goals while others do not?*

Let me first clarify my definition of "achievement." Achievement is reaching a level of success based on a specific or general goal you have set. It is not based on society's interpretation of achievement, but on your own. The creation of realistic goals for personal achievement allows for better living, and I believe we all deserve to live better.

If you're reading this book, you're probably more concerned with ridding yourself of negative patterns, than with reinforcing positive ones. It's important to recognize that you have both. The areas of your life that are going smoothly do not consume as much attention as those that are not going well.

Working on yourself so that you can achieve meaningful goals and have the life you want isn't easy. Negative or undermining patterns can be deeply ingrained and hard to overcome. You need both motivation and discipline for the task. But to rid yourself of negative patterns, you must first be willing to look unflinchingly at yourself.

Be your own toughest critic and your own most enthusiastic supporter. Remember and draw strength and self-esteem from your successes in life, however minor they might seem to you. By consciously establishing some islands of competence, you give yourself the necessary confidence to take on greater challenges.

Where Will Change Take You?

In *Breaking the Pattern,* the objective is not necessarily to help you get rich or to make you feel blissfully good about yourself every waking moment, but rather to help you define and set your goals, and then show you how to work effectively to achieve them. If the byproduct of *Breaking the Pattern* is that you get rich and are joyful all the time, it's a bonus.

But I can tell you from firsthand experience, there's no magic formula or quick fix. Nor is this book a recipe for success for which you just add water and stir. If you think something will jump off the pages of this book and change you without your own committed input, don't walk, but run back to the bookstore and get your money back. However, this book will give you the essential ingredients and strategies for breaking negative patterns, and for defining and achieving your individual goals. *Breaking the Pattern* will not do all the work for you. That's something you have to do for yourself. But first, you have to believe that *you are worth it.*

To do so, you should be willing to overcome what I call the "Corniness Factor." The information and suggestions in this book range from the scientific to the "corny." I'll be asking you to make declaratory statements like, "I am going to change my life and achieve my goals." It sounds exaggerated, overly simplistic, and sophomoric, if not completely uncomfortable. But in researching this book, I was continually surprised by how many successful individuals—many of whom I've interviewed, including artists, writers, chefs, directors, CEOs, people who have lost weight, quit smoking, and improved their lives—used this statement as a starting strategy for personal achievement and breaking patterns.

I can assure you that the successful people in your life who you admire apply many, or all, of the techniques described in this book. *Success is no accident, nor is it unconscious.* People who achieve their goals are almost always acutely aware of what directions they take in reaching their destinations. They also use very specific techniques, which I'll ask you to implement. In order to change your life, *you have to be serious and committed to self-discovery and self-growth.*

Rather than take responsibility for what happens to us—or even how we react to the events in our lives—it seems easier to make excuses or blame others (or even destiny) for what we have and who we are. Individual responsibility and control of your life don't stem from dodging or avoiding difficulties, but from strategizing and coping with the difficulties that come your way. Nobody's life is free of obstacles, conflict, and struggle. As unpleasant as it appears, conflict forces us to make decisions, shaping and strengthening character along the way.

These ideas on personal responsibility led me to another realization: *We may not be fully responsible for every event in our lives; accidents do happen, both lucky and unlucky ones. However, we are solely responsible for how we respond to these events, and how we allow these events to shape us. Many of our own patterns—which we are in control of—bring us opportunity, success, and failure.*

To break patterns, we must recognize them as our own creations and transform them through concentrated goal setting, discipline, perseverance, and achievement. This book will walk you through these Principles step-by-step.

Beginning the Journey

As a result of plenty of hard work and applying the five Principles in this book, I was able to overcome one of my patterns: choosing terrible business partners. I was able to find a great partner by observing and looking for good qualities that would accentuate my own talents. I teamed up and co-founded a communications company, a forerunner in multimedia development that created online entertainment and original programming. More than 700 magazines, newspapers, and broadcasts recognized the company's success.

Secondly, I was able to overcome my uncanny ability to meet the most inappropriate and incompatible women, many of whom had destructive personalities and were all wrong for me. I had repeated this negative pattern since the time I started dating. I finally met a woman who was not the slightest bit destructive—the woman I married. Shannon has helped me become a better person, a state of being I really didn't think was possible just a few years ago.

I take pride in these accomplishments, but what I consider one of my most rewarding and difficult patterns to overcome was being overweight. I have been on any and every diet as far back as I can remember. You name it: high protein, high fat, grapefruit, no fruit. Each dieting experience ended in dismal failure. Once I understood my eating patterns and could apply the five Principles, I was able to lose the weight and keep it off. The weight has remained off for six years now.

As a result of my success and struggle with weight loss, I founded a company devoted to nutrition and fitness, which features weight-loss coaching using email. With this company, the objective is to pass along to others around the world the information and knowledge I have both synthesized and used to succeed. To date, not only have we counseled thousands of people and helped them achieve their weight loss goals, but the site was voted one of *Forbes* magazine's "Best of the Web" and *Health* magazine's "Top 25 Web Sites For Women."

My goal in *Breaking the Pattern* is not to preach, not to give complicated, idealistic "cheerleader" instructions, but instead to provide practical, simple, and concise steps to help you take control of your life by recognizing and breaking patterns. As you become aware of the patterns that prevent you from being a success, either personally or professionally—and take responsibility for how they affect the way you live—you will begin to live a more fruitful and happier life. It's a profoundly liberating experience to recognize these patterns and to realize you can break free of them.

We are all, largely, the authors of our own lives, and we can write a different outcome than the one we seem to be headed for.

I believe you can do it.

Charles S. Platkin
New York, NY

PATTERNS
FAILURE
RESPONSIBILITY
GOALS
ACHIEVEMENT

CHAPTER • ONE

What's a Pattern and How Do I Know What Mine Are?

. . . and once again she shuddered with the evidence that time was not passing, but that it was turning in a circle.
—Gabriel García Márquez, *One Hundred Years of Solitude*

The definition of insanity is repeating the same thing again and again and expecting a different outcome.
—Anonymous

Have you ever had a sickening sense of reliving the same events in your life—of even having the same conversations or arguments—again and again? Relationships, jobs, or projects may begin full of hope, but somehow, they don't work out for you. You sense a common theme—the endings and the feelings after each mishap or failure are so familiar. You feel that people are always letting you down, betraying you, demanding too much of you, not giving back what you deserve or that you just can't catch a break. Most of all, every new experience or relationship *feels familiar, as if it happened before and you didn't like it the first time around.* These experiences are the result of your patterns.

Patterns emerge everywhere, in nature and in life. Patterns bring structure to the universe and give it order. They're present in either the

3

smallest bits or greatest masses of matter. A pattern may be held in place by electrons circling a nucleus or planets revolving around the sun. Patterns are present in our genes, in our cultures, and in the history of our nations. Patterns play an important role in our psychological makeup, personality, and behavior. Jobs and relationships travel familiar paths—and we often feel as if we're going in circles.

This sense of life as a recurring pattern might seem confining at first. If you're trapped in a never-ending circle, what's the use of even trying? But the realization that your life might have certain patterns, and that you have the ability to recognize and modify them, will liberate you. Life doesn't have to be chaotic.

Awareness need not breed gloom or doom. This is one of the most important ideas to remember and take with you through this book. I firmly believe that even in your darkest moments, golden opportunities for insight, reflection, and real change present themselves. In fact, often these are the most suitable times for growth. It's unfortunate, but true: we do more self-improvement when we're "down-and-out" then when we're happy and peppy. These moments are the biggest opportunity for a breakthrough: When something is not working in your life, why not dig in to find the pattern(s) of behavior underlying your disappointments? Never mind what others may do and say. Only you can change your life.

You might think:

▸ "Why bother looking back at all? Why would I want to do that. I should let it go, move on."
▸ "What could I learn? I've tried my best—I'm done."
▸ "I can't control other people, especially when they've got the power. Give me power and I'll show what I can do—things will be different, you'll see."
▸ "I just need one lucky break . . ."

- "My life is already mapped out for me; this is my destiny."
- "I guess I'm just unlucky—what can I tell you?"
- Or perhaps, "Things are okay . . . I'm just going through a rough time."

You will not find the answer by ignoring the past or by being "strong." The real answer lies in a willingness to ask yourself these questions:

- How am I contributing to my own misery, disappointments, unhappiness, setbacks, or lack of achievement?
- Do I really have choices?
- What patterns am I repeating so that I wind up in the same place no matter how different my starting point?

If nothing else, consider this: What harm could come from considering these questions? Not much—and actually, this is the first step toward improving your life. When you become aware of where your own personal patterns of behavior lead you, and then modify them, your life will change. Remember: You have to be conscious of how you act. You cannot change what you are not aware of, or what you are not willing to accept.

This Principle is about discovering the patterns that underlie the areas of your life that you find less than satisfying, as well as taking the first step toward changing them in thought and action. That familiar sickening feeling in your stomach is an invitation to start thinking straight. Be grateful for it! When you notice a wrenching knot in your gut, it usually means something's not right. Working through this step can begin to transform your life, but only if you have the courage to dig deeper and dare to change.

However, let me caution you. Although I am recommending that you look at yourself unflinchingly and unsparingly, you have to forgive yourself for falling into patterns, even as you vow to get to the bottom of them and change the destructive ones. The solutions to your problems are often the best ones you *think* you have available to you at that time. No one consciously tries to come up with self-destructive, self-sabotaging behavior, but many times you are hindered by what feels like a lack of options because you have developed patterns that closed off other possibilities. Leaving patterns unexamined will only compound your problems.

In order to break your patterns, you need to find new ways of looking at the same problem. If you have trouble getting to a particular place with your car, you don't need a new car—you may just need a new map. Making a new map may require throwing out or destroying the old to avoid the temptation of falling back on it or of using it as a shortcut. Think about how you get to work each day. You once needed a map or someone to guide the way. Now, you get there without thinking about it. But what happens when your usual route is under construction and there is a detour? You need to be innovative, creative, and thoughtful in calling upon the resources available to you to find the most efficient path to your destination.

Think of yourself as both the driver and the car in your life. Occasionally, the road you travel is unexpectedly bumpy or dangerous, there might be roadblocks or the road simply might not exist. Kicking the car in frustration or damning the person or job you were traveling to, doesn't get you back on the road and into gear. What does get you on the right road again is adaptation to circumstances and the process of creating a new map. What gets you what you want is your flexibility; your ability to change.

Continuing on the same course, perpetuating negative patterns no matter how unsatisfying, numbing, or even destructive they may be, occurs because it feels safe, familiar, comfortable and convenient. No wonder it's so hard to change!

Can a Leopard Really Change Its Spots?

What should you know about change? What is it?

The dictionary describes change as: 1. to make different. 2. to exchange for something else. The synonyms for change are: alter, modify, transform, vary.

Perhaps you've wondered: Is anyone really helped by the self-help industry, or are the forces of genetics and the circumstances of one's life too strong for any person to radically change? Certainly, for all the self-help material around for so many decades, all too many people continue to lead lives full of yearning and, sometimes, searing desperation.

It's important to recognize that there are certain qualities about you that are permanent and unchanging. You cannot, no matter how disciplined or determined you are, for instance, change your race or parentage or cultural heritage. Increasing evidence suggests that temperaments are set at a very early age and that this fundamental part of your being accompanies you throughout life. But this doesn't mean that being shy or extroverted when you're young cannot be modified to help you get what you want later in life.

Change is definitely possible, despite centuries of the dominant idea that life is pre-determined, wholly defined by forces beyond your control, and outside of you. You are not merely created, but also a creator, and your biggest creation is yourself. I know this is true because I've been able to change my life in radical ways by using the strategies in this book. I have heard stories of success and failure that have further convinced me of how a clear mind and a determined outlook can change nearly anyone for the better. A few years after writing that letter to my friend, my life and work improved drastically. I'm involved in the most fulfilling relationship of my life with a wonderful woman. I have a successful weight-loss counseling business. And, I have never been happier with the way I look and feel.

But some kinds of change are clearly and more easily possible. I've collected an enormous amount of evidence to support my belief that you can alter your life's course. There are some very specific and highly useful methods that give you the opportunity to achieve what you set out to do, within your own limitations, but beyond your expectations. Psychologist David C. McClelland, formerly at Harvard and Wesleyan and now based at Boston University, specializes in the study of human motivation. His views have evolved from the basic Freudian idea that motivation and personality are formed early in childhood and never change, to the view that human motivation can be modified in adulthood.

McClelland devised an achievement/motivation training course that took as its starting point this assumption: If you are taught to think, talk, and act like a high-achiever, then you will actually achieve more. He began this course in India, using untrained businessmen as his model group. He found that the trainees he worked with were more likely to engage in subsequent entrepreneurial activity than non-trainees. In other words, his thesis about motivation was correct.

Recurring Events, Patterns, and Familiarities

Psychologists tell us that we establish patterns of coping, succeeding, and failing early in life. The relationships you had with your parents when you were a child largely determine how you relate to the world for the rest of your life. If you're not conscious of how these relationships work as an adult, you continue to act and react the same ways, whether or not your actions get you what you want. For example, a child who's physically or verbally abused by a parent may simply block out the experience as a way of dealing with pain. For a child with limited coping capabilities, this may be the most adaptive strategy available. But if denial becomes an ingrained pattern, the inner abused child is still controlling the actions and reactions of the adult, who may not recognize other available strategies. In some cases, the common solution for deadening pain in childhood, like living in denial, may itself become the problem later in life.

What happens?

One complication of denying unpleasant situations and not confronting problems or crises is that you stay stuck in the past. I recently counseled a woman with a weight problem. Betty ate compulsively whenever she was frustrated or depressed. She'd tried many diets, and would often end up blaming herself for not losing weight and keeping it off. More frequently, she'd blame the diet.

When I met with Betty, she told me that she couldn't "dwell on" why she overate—she simply wanted to lose the weight quickly. She said, "Just give me a simple diet to follow—that's *all* I need." That's actually the last thing Betty needed to lose weight effectively and permanently. She already knew almost everything about healthy eating. First, Betty needed to understand why she ate when she was depressed and frustrated, and *who or what she blamed for her being overweight.*

Awareness of your patterns, and what causes them to perpetuate, is a crucial first step to changing. You are the author of your own life—you are the creator of your patterns—therefore you can change them. *Life patterns have a funny way of creating a momentum that is difficult to alter.* You need to take control of your patterns, and not let your patterns control you. Betty needed to find out why she was choosing to be overweight.

You are what you choose to be.

Betty was making a choice to be fat. She was choosing food over her desire to look better and live a healthier lifestyle.

Patterns and What They Mean to You

What do I mean by *pattern of behavior?* Let me begin with a definition. The dictionary says a pattern is: 1. a mode of behavior regarded as characteristic of persons or things or 2. an original or model considered for or deserving of imitation. As conscious, creative beings, we experience both.

We're all creatures of what I call *patterns.* From waking up to getting dressed to simply talking to a friend, we've learned to do things a certain way. You may not even be aware of, for example, how you get dressed in the morning. Do you put on your shirt first? Or your socks? Where did you learn to do this? If you were told to change the order of which item of clothing you put on first or last, you could. But before you switch from automatic to the optional setting, you have to become aware of what you do *without* thinking. To permanently change you might need a reminder every morning, such as a note on your closet door—perhaps, until the new system becomes a pattern.

Not every aspect of life needs to be examined and held up to scrutiny. It is useful to do some of life's more mundane tasks, such as getting dressed, somewhat automatically and without too much thought. But what if it became clear that your way of getting dressed was causing you problems? Or, a more likely example, what if you discovered that your diet was causing you profound health problems? People who experience this, report having to learn how to eat all over again; hardly an easy task for an adult to undertake. But when it is a matter of survival (seven major diseases are caused by being overweight), many people are able to change fundamental aspects of their behavior.

Your negative psychological patterns are much more complex and insidious than mundane patterns such as how we eat cereal, put on socks or carve a chicken. Patterns are a series of interconnected decision-making processes, the result of how your mind frames your experiences, usually formed in early childhood. Your patterns of loving and choosing partners are almost always influenced by your family relationships. Your ambitions and professional desires are often affected by your school experiences or how people reacted to your efforts in childhood.

Which patterns keep you from moving ahead? The following anecdotes illustrate the six most common undermining patterns and how to understand them. Do you recognize yourself in any of these?

- Finding someone/something to blame
- Self-sabotaging and self-paralyzing behavior
- Bad choices compounded by denial
- Always seeking the short cut and the path of least resistance
- Choosing to be overweight
- Substance abuse

Which one(s) most relate to who you are?

Of all the negative patterns I've seen in people and experienced personally, none is more common and unproductive than blaming others (or events/money/timing, etc.) for our failures and disappointments in life. We may think, "Well, if I can avoid getting mixed up with that person again, then I'll be happy/win/get the promotion I deserve/find love . . ."

What's blaming about? It makes us feel better—and gives us an out—but this solution is only temporary. What blaming really does is blind us to the root of our problems, making us feel more helpless in the long run.

Gary is an example of a blamer who is confused about the kind of choices he can make—and remember Gary does have choices.

When he was fresh out of college, Gary decided to start his own business. He'd worked at an auto body shop through school and figured he knew enough about the business to open his own place. He had the desire and the smarts, but not the capital. He needed someone to help finance the business. He met Jake, who expressed genuine interest in Gary's venture. He arranged a meeting with Jake, who had the qualities Gary was looking for: money and the personality for this kind of business—which meant Jake was outgoing and socially at ease, unlike him.

Jake showed up an hour late for their first meeting—in fact, Jake showed up late for every meeting Gary set up. He always seemed to forget, or would lose, Gary's telephone number. When they got down to business, Jake boasted about how good he was at avoiding collection agents. Despite these worrisome signs, Gary still liked (or needed) Jake and decided they'd make the perfect team. He simply convinced himself it would all work out. "I thought Jake would work out well enough," Gary said. "I'm sure Jake will be an excellent compliment to the business, and besides I need him to get the financial backing for the business. I'll let the other stuff slide."

Their auto body shop opened. Business was good, except for one problem: Jake still acted, Gary said, "like Jake pre-partnership." He was always late, forgot key meetings, neglected to pay important bills, and was generally irresponsible. Jake's lateness often lost them customers. After two years, Gary was losing money despite all his best efforts. Gary finally sold his half of the shop and decided to start over.

Gary figured the auto body shop was the wrong business for him, and that Jake was the wrong partner, so he decided to start another business. This time he would try selling insurance. Again, he needed capital so he sought out and chose another partner, Steve. He was a little demanding and rough around the edges, but to balance them out, Steve was also punctual, responsible and outgoing. Gary felt he had made a good deal. Two years later, Gary was in the same situation as before. "Business started off well, then something went amiss. I underestimated Steve's 'rough edges,'" Gary said. "It got us into trouble." Apparently, Steve's abrasive and controlling style alienated clients, employees, and eventually even Gary. The bottom line: They were losing money. Gary blamed Steve's grating behavior for turning away clients and eventually sinking the business.

Gary tried again, this time, starting an Internet site and getting in on the cutting edge of new technology. He still felt uncomfortable doing it alone. Because he had little capital, Gary needed someone who could build the technology in exchange for equity in the company. This time, he chose Bob for a partner, a computer expert whose personality was very unassuming, "nerdy," and quiet. Bob was also not driven to work very hard for the business and usually spent his days surfing the Web rather than building out the Web site. "A year later," Gary told me, "I was looking at another problem business that still hadn't made any money." He blamed Bob; he blamed the Internet; he blamed the government for their regulations; he blamed the failure of the Asian economies on undermining his expansion plans. Gary blamed everyone and everything but himself.

Understanding the Blame Game

The fact is, there is no one more responsible for the way your life works out than you. For every move you make, you have choices. This doesn't mean other people won't influence you and have a profound impact on how you think, feel, or act. Starting with your parents, many people affect you in great and small ways. However, after hundreds of interviews, I confirmed that one of the key characteristics of *all* successful people is their ability to avoid the trap of blaming others for whatever failures or setbacks trip them up along the road to achievement. Blaming others means there's nothing within your power or control to fix a problem. It means there are no choices. If successful people bought into believing their lives were not in their control, it would force them to acknowledge defeat. No successful person would ever tolerate this kind of surrendering to the whims of others. There's a big difference between taking responsibility for one's life (being accountable to yourself) and self-blame (believing everything is your fault). The first is empowering and propels you forward; the second is counter-productive, depressing, and a futile exercise in beating yourself up. Remember: Blaming yourself is as destructive as blaming someone or something else for your own misguided efforts.

Successful recognition comes from carefully examining your patterns, not placing blame on anyone or anything, but instead, looking for motivations underlying those mistakes in order to correct them in the future.

Holding others responsible for your failures or successes plants you on the road to helplessness. You can't change other people, you can only change yourself and the way you relate and respond to people. To change your patterns, you need to find out what motivated you to **use blame***, what you get out of it, and set out to consciously become accountable for your actions and your feelings.*

Here's what happened to Gary:

Gary did not acknowledge his pattern of picking bad business partners, ignoring the warning signs, and not taking responsibility for the results of his choices. When I met Gary, he told me about his three situations, and he was confused about why each relationship ended badly. I was frank with him. I shared with him some of the Principles I was developing. At my suggestion, he sat down and reflected on his experiences, writing down the positive and negative sides of each of his business situations. He then could begin to answer his own question of *why* he did what he did. Basically, by not learning effectively from his failures, he repeated them. He depended solely on others, and those others were wrong for him.

Gary realized that he'd selected each of his partners in haste, and specifically, because he was afraid to fail, not succeed, on his own. By taking partners, he always had someone to blame when things went wrong. Gary also chose to ignore all of the signs pointing to the faults of his partners. He justified his decisions by saying they provided what he needed at the time, whether it was capital, personality, or expertise.

Eventually Gary decided that if he wanted to start his own business, he'd have to finance it himself. He took a job with a big consulting firm, and worked his heart out for two years to save enough start-up money. Working for someone else wasn't his ideal situation, but he realized that it was a necessary sacrifice to create what he wanted. He soon banked enough to start his own business, another auto body shop. The business took off.

Gary knows he's on the right path. Before this, he'd chosen the wrong way to go about being in business. Now, he understands the concept of mastering one's own ship and being responsible—and is enjoying the freedom that breaking his blaming pattern has given him.

Self-Sabotaging and Self-Paralyzing Behavior

This is a big category, since self-sabotage takes many different forms including a *lack of follow-through*, and, on the other end of the scale, a misguided idea of *perfectionism*.

A lack of follow-through implies that there's energy put into the planning stages, but a real paucity of commitment in getting the job done. Perfectionists, however, may have follow-through, but at the same time, demand high or unrealistic standards that may never be met—nothing and no one is ever good enough. Perfectionists have a hard time letting things go or saying, "This is finished. I did my best!"

Sam, a 50-year-old New Yorker, embodies this pattern.

A gifted writer, Sam had been hired at a variety of newspapers and magazines throughout his career, but every job ended in frustration for him and his employer. Sam was a very hard worker who diligently put in long hours to produce great stories. The problem was that Sam always missed his deadlines, and consistently argued that he was not given sufficient time to finish. Sam refused to learn how to use a computer, which made things easier to correct and print out and insisted on using an outdated typewriter. To add to his self-perpetuating burdens, Sam would not allow a researcher to help him gather facts or conduct interviews. Instead, he went to the library to do it "the right way." The perfect way. He was fired.

Sam had the credentials and enough personality to get another job as an editor at a local newspaper. Again, he worked long hours, always trying to make every story and column "perfect," thereby neglecting his other duties. He would edit and re-edit stories, causing the paper to pay huge late fees to printers. Many subscribers canceled subscriptions because the paper came out late. Finally, Sam was fired. He blamed the paper's "lack of journalistic integrity," not his inadequate work patterns and time-wasting perfectionism, for his termination.

Rather than trying to learn why he was having such trouble, Sam continued bouncing from job to job, never understanding his pattern. Predictably, Sam continuously felt misunderstood and undervalued. Many times, he feared his writing wasn't good enough. Now in his 50s with no savings, few assets, and even fewer career choices, Sam worries if his big break will ever come his way. He has the nagging feeling that he won't live up to his potential, or, as he puts it in basketball terms, "I might never quite 'drive to the basket.'"

Understanding Self-Sabotage and Self-Paralyzing Behavior

Sam makes creative choices that exacerbate his problems and practical career choices that sabotage him financially. Most of all, he looks everywhere except at himself for answers and solutions. Sam needs to ask himself *why he chose not to reach his goal of becoming a great writer.*

At a deeper level, he simply does not believe he's worthy of happiness or that he's good enough to succeed (fear of failing). This lack of self-confidence and a pattern of perfectionism keeps him spinning his wheels. Perfectionists like Sam set unrealistic high goals or standards, pursue them compulsively, yet derive very little pleasure from their efforts. They soon see the chinks and cracks in what they thought might be perfect, whether it's a relationship, a job, or how they regard themselves. Perfectionists think in extremes and even a minor failure, to them, is a sign of complete personal failure. They live in what therapists call "a tyranny of shoulds."

Sam sabotages his success by laboring over newspaper writing, which demands speed and accuracy. He wants stroking and acclaim for his artistic and diligent work, but he doesn't get it. Sam used his time at the newspaper to avoid facing reality. If Sam continues to sabotage and paralyze his career by not putting himself in a situation where his talents can be tested, then he never has to find out if he would be successful as an artistic and creative writer. He continually chooses to live under an illusion, instead of really finding the most appropriate place to work. Sam has always had a number of career choices, some obvious and some not so obvious. Maybe he shouldn't have been writing for newspapers at all, or, maybe he shouldn't have hoped to be viewed as a respected artist in workplaces where artistry was unimportant. Perhaps he should have been happy with his "day job," and just gotten through with it, come home and done his own creative writing at his own pace.

Sam continued to focus on losing his jobs, and wondered what was wrong with the newspaper or his writing. Rather than utilizing his mistakes and failures to propel him forward productively, he wasted energy on regret and reliving each failure. If we were all rational creatures all the time, we'd strive for goals without playing games with ourselves and jeopardizing our chances for success. Conversely, some of us try to fail, even those with a more pronounced need for achievement. I, too, have been guilty of self-paralyzing behavior. In college, I always tried to master as many different skills as possible. I fooled myself into believing I could turn myself into a real competitor in the world, in any field.

By trying to overachieve, I had a ready-made excuse for failing in fifteen different areas. This way, I could give myself the excuse, "Well, with so many balls in the air, it had to be difficult to focus all my attention on *that one thing.*" Whatever that may be. Then again, by splitting my attention into many different projects, I felt as if I had many chances to succeed. I could hedge my bets. The same amount of energy put into one solid area could have produced rewarding results. I was afraid of failing, and if I focused on just one thing, and I failed, the failure would be right in my face. As a result, I kept myself from succeeding at anything at all.

Bad Choices Compounded by Denial

Although she never admits to it, Amanda always had doubt about the institution of marriage. Her parents had been miserable together. While they were each interesting and vibrant alone, as a couple, they were intolerably bitter. When she was in her early teens, her mother abandoned the family to run off with another man. Her father, a brilliant but selfish man, had very little time for Amanda or her sisters, and let them know they were on their own once they turned 18.

Throughout her 20s and 30s, Amanda had a series of relationships with interesting but unstable men. Many of them were involved in the music industry or were ambitious Wall Streeters. It wasn't unusual for her latest boyfriend to have a substance abuse or drinking problem. "Until the bad times, I had a good time with most of them," she said, "and pretty much told myself a guy could be entertaining until the real thing came along."

Although she wasn't much interested in marriage, Amanda was still deeply hurt when these relationships ended, feeling rejected when men she really didn't want to marry turned out not to want to marry her. She shouldn't have been surprised. Many of these men told her from the start that they were uninterested in marriage—but she secretly hoped they would change if they fell in love.

As each relationship neared the break-up point, Amanda clung to any glimmer of hope for as long as possible. "I heard myself promising some guy who just said he didn't want me that I'd be willing to change," she told me. "I'd ask him what he needed from me in order to love me. What was I doing that I could change? The guys inevitably left me, and both of us felt bad." Predictably, Amanda was devastated by the loss, and angry, once again, about having her fragile ego wounded. Now in her late 30s, Amanda is cynical about what men can give emotionally, and about her long-term possibilities for romantic love. She wonders, "Are there any good men out there, or am I destined to be alone forever?"

Understanding Bad Choices Compounded by Denial

If blame makes us helpless, denial paralyzes us. Denial is refusing to acknowledge and act upon the warning signs that something is terribly wrong and about to cause us harm, loss, or emotional pain. Gary ("The Blamer") ignored the obvious signs that potential partners were irresponsible, immature, or irrational men. He excused their weaknesses, hoping that things would just somehow work themselves out. Likewise, Amanda ("The Denier") couldn't face the fact that she chose men who would not care about her, and heard only what she wanted to hear. Furthermore, she completely denied her own ambivalence and doubts about maintaining a successful long-term relationship.

People who enter destructive relationships often ignore signals that tell them they're getting involved with an overly possessive/irrationally jealous/coldly detached/potentially violent mate/partner/employer (as did Gary and Amanda). Job seekers sometimes ignore the telltale clues during an interview that a boss or the corporate culture may be a potential nightmare. For example, knowing that the company's employees are nervous or scared about losing their jobs or, a telling comment that the management clearly doesn't recognize the needs of its employees.

If you burrow too deeply into denial, you place yourself in great emotional, and even physical, jeopardy. Experts say that the most important facets of someone's personality are revealed within the first six weeks of a relationship—if you really pay attention and remain fully aware during this time, you'll see everything you need to see. Amanda, for one, *saw but did not act.*

A recent study shows you can predict the success of a marriage by listening to a couple's first few arguments. It's not only what they argue about, but also how they argue and where the argument takes them. When you argue in denial, you can't hear what's really going on, and the argument is repeated again and again in a mind-numbing manner. So we often see things, but choose to ignore their existence or repress them for our own purposes—a dangerous and destructive pattern.

Usually, denial arises out of desperation, as with Amanda. She knew right from the start, deep in her heart, that the men she chose were not right for her. She made a choice to ignore the warning signs—it made life easier for her. She most probably was afraid of being in a long-term relationship, afraid of getting hurt. In reality, Amanda, or any of you, cannot afford not to act. Think about it. Have you ever had a sneaking suspicion that a relationship would not work out or that a business opportunity was too good to be true from the very start? And did your feelings or your "gut instinct" get it right even though you went along for the ride?

Denial can become a pernicious pattern, a way of getting by in difficult circumstances and avoiding confrontations. Invariably, those who practice denial repeat the same mistakes again and again, and the end result gets worse and worse. But when you *break the pattern*, you figure out what you're denying and why. You may find that the general, vague anxiety you feel is lifted once you pinpoint your fears.

Always Seeking the Short Cut and the Path of Least Resistance

Eric, a 32-year-old man from Connecticut, touts himself as highly motivated to become a "success." As he puts it, "I'm willing to do what it takes." His goal is to be independently wealthy by investing in real estate.

Eric has another goal: He doesn't want to answer to anyone, so working for a real estate company to learn everything he can is out of the question. Instead, he spends most of his free time studying for and planning his real estate fortune to give Donald Trump a run for his money. To prove how serious he is, he continues to buy many "Get rich quick in real estate" tapes and videos that he sees advertised on late-night TV.

After a few years of working as an assistant manager in a mall-based candy store, and living hand-to-mouth, Eric finally woke up to the fact that he didn't have enough cash to buy property. One day, he lost hope. But first, he felt angry and cheated by everyone and everything, including the late night get-rich gurus who promised him overnight success. On a tear, he dumped his real estate tapes and videos into the trash when he thought he found a better, faster answer: going into the phone up 900-number business. That didn't bring him his fortune either. He then switched to enrolling in one multi-level marketing scheme after another, always in pursuit of his dream of attaining great wealth.

What's interesting about Eric is that he's not a fool. He really *does* have the potential to be a success, but he refuses to focus on one career goal and put in the time and effort to work his way upward. He thinks like a Las Vegas weekend gambler or the person who drops his last $100 on lottery tickets every Friday payday. He wants a miracle on the path of least resistance.

I'm not saying that you shouldn't think outside of the box or create new opportunities, but get-rich-quick schemes tend to make very few people rich other than the person who thought up scheme in the first place. What Eric needs to succeed is a long-range plan to work in real estate, perhaps a job within the industry to get a feel for it and to develop relationships. Eventually, he'll figure out how to own and sell property.

Understanding Short Cuts and the Path of Least Resistance

Sometimes it feels easier (and a whole lot less painful) to take the first thing that comes along. Business executives often hire people who are not up to par or who don't share the same commitment, and then become increasingly resentful when they shoulder more and more of the work. On the employee side, you may take a job that's unchallenging or unsuitable, just for the sake of security. At another level, you may settle for unchallenging or unsuitable because that's what was offered, never daring to negotiate for anything better. And you may also act out the same pattern of taking short cuts in your romantic life—willing to unconsciously settle for someone who is "not the one" to avoid your fear of being alone.

Too much passive acceptance fuels low self-esteem. Of the thousands of people I've read about, interviewed, and counseled, I have heard many versions of the same complaint, "This is my life and there's nothing I can do." Most of them seethe with frustration and resentment, but are afraid to fight, to dream, to dare, or to really "go for it." The world does a good enough job of placing limits on us in hundreds of small ways, and we don't need to collaborate, agree, or surrender. At the same time, we shouldn't fool ourselves into thinking, as Eric did, that "life will hand you" a shortcut to success, achievement, and happiness.

Choosing to be Overweight

Everyone wants to be healthier, more fit, and attractive. For some, the pursuit of health and beauty is an all-consuming drive. For others, it seems like being physically fit is a prerequisite to happiness. Because our patterns of eating and exercising are so deeply ingrained, they can be some of the more difficult patterns to break.

Overeating is common in so many of our lives. Currently, more than 50 percent of the American population is overweight, and that number increases every day. Of particular interest is the "yo-yo" dieting behavior of people who are trying desperately to lose weight, and are willing to do almost anything to shed those unwanted pounds.

Given the small exception of those people with temporary or permanent medical issues, I'd say that *breaking the patterns* that go hand-in-hand with being overweight, including battling with negative self-image and unhealthy diets, is truly possible by applying the principles from this book.

Not only do I counsel people every day on weight loss, but I also know from years of personal experience that to actually lose weight, you must change your behavior. I also know that breaking the "fat" pattern is impossible unless you begin with this simple first step: make a choice to lose weight, and then keep your goal in sight and in your consciousness all the time. Remember: It's the little things that can trip you up, such as snacking on popcorn or candy at the movies or sitting in front of the television with a pint of ice cream. You need to always be conscious of *why you want to lose weight.* Ask yourself before indulging: What is the payoff to being in good shape? Be clear about your goal. In order to overcome one desire, like overeating, it helps to replace it with another desire—a desire which is stronger, more potent, and clear.

When attempting any type of change, you don't just want to move away from the negative pattern—it's simply not enough. When you move away from a negative pattern, you reduce the pain it causes you. For example, if you start losing weight, you will feel better, and the pain from being overweight will be reduced. As the pain subsides, you will be more likely to go back to where you started—eating again, and gaining the weight back. To avoid this pattern, make sure that you move toward something, instead of away from it. This is where goal setting becomes important.

For me, it was my desire to change my appearance, and avoid getting diabetes, a disease that runs in my family. You're battling your own demanding hungry demons, and they are unrelenting. Make the choice to *lose weight and be fit.* Your life may depend on it.

Alcohol and Substance Abuse

Like overeating, addiction to anything is a deeply entrenched pattern of behavior—it's a destructive way of coping with the difficulties life sometimes tosses at us. The old-fashioned view maintains that alcoholism and other addictions to controlled substances result from some moral weakness, some failure of will. Today, many researchers believe there is a biological component to certain kinds of addiction, and to that extent, such addictive patterns may be difficult to break without medical help.

Understanding Alcohol and Substance Abuse

Few believe that the solution to an addiction resides solely in popping a magic pill that will make the craving go away. Others are convinced that isolation from the stuff kicks the habit. The truth lies somewhere in the middle. The addiction is about the addict's habit. No matter how much medical treatment he or she gets, the addict can't truly recover without recognizing and correcting the behavioral patterns that either created or worsen the problem. Roughly 60 percent of alcoholics relapse within three months of getting treatment, and according to one study, 76 percent of cocaine users return to the drug in the same short time span. Psychologist Emil Chiauzzi, in an attempt to understand the reasons behind these statistics, studied 90 relapsed addicts dependent on a variety of drugs, particularly alcohol, cocaine, and marijuana. Despite the fact that they all attended support groups, he found they "harbored misconceptions, misunderstandings, and just plain wrong information about themselves and what causes people to resume their addictions—errors that put them at greater risk of doing just that." He noted three personality traits typical of addicts:

> ▶ **Dependency**: Addicts who aren't accountable for their addiction haven't taken the crucial first step in the hard emotional work involved in recovery. Rather than face up to what they're doing to themselves, they lean on alcohol or drugs.

▸ **Passive-Aggressive Tendencies**: Rather than being accountable for his/her own actions and situation, the addict directs his/her anger and blame at others. Passive-aggressive people tend to procrastinate, manipulate others, and feel victimized even when they are doing the victimizing.

▸ **Narcissism**: This describes the inability to take and accept feedback from others, no matter how intelligent and accurate it may be. Narcissists tend to overestimate their own progress and lack true self-knowledge.

Many addicts substitute one addiction for another. To replace the high that drugs offer, some immerse themselves in work. After putting in 100 hours a week, stressed-out workaholics are likely to turn to their drug of choice to alleviate fatigue and anxiety. Others might enter addictive relationships in which they expect their partners to solve all their problems. But temporary solutions only lead to a false sense of security.

Those who equate abstinence or attending AA meetings with recovery end up with a limited view of recovery—this ends up being a weak spot for many addicts. What they really need is personal growth and an opportunity to develop feelings of self-worth. As Chiauzzi notes, "Those who have the most successful recoveries also learn the importance of understanding themselves."

Many addicts fail to spot the warning signs that a relapse is imminent. These signs include a desire to spend time with drug-using friends, mood swings that include depression or irritability, poor physical functioning, and a loss of structure in daily routines. Even if an addict relapses, it doesn't mean that he or she is doomed forever and should stop trying. As long as people are alive, they're capable of changing for the better.

Progress may be followed by a setback, but setbacks merely send us back to the drawing board. It's important to understand addictive behaviors because it can give us clues to overcoming the negative patterns in our own lives—we all have certain behaviors or habits we have trouble overcoming.

No matter what kind of destructive pattern or behavior people may be engaged in, they have the ability, within themselves—and with a great deal of work and support—to overcome them and lead better, more fulfilling lives.

Trigger Events and Motivation

Changing patterns that are almost reflexive and automatic is hard and sometimes painful work. And like most self-betterment, it takes a great deal of motivation. There is usually something or someone—a situation, event, or individual—that motivates you to change. This event or series of events makes you realize that you want to change—that you need to change. A trigger event can be a humiliating personal disaster, like an upstanding citizen who's arrested for stealing to feed a big-time, hidden drug habit. A trigger can be an invitation to a reunion, which motivates you to get in the best shape to impress people who haven't seen you in a long time.

Triggers can be as clear as getting fired or ending an important relationship. In a Hollywood movie, it's called the "inciting incident": the event or situation that causes the heroine to "wake up and smell the coffee." This is when she realizes she is just "no good," she has been drinking too much, not treating a spouse well, ignoring her child, and so on. That splash of ice water on the face—that's the trigger. A trigger can be a much quieter affair than something that hits you over the head. It may be a casual but hurtful comment about your appearance or status. Common triggers include birthdays, anniversaries, New Year's Eve, the holidays, or any other significant event that makes us reflect on where we've been and where we're going.

Don't ignore any trigger, no matter how small, because it's a sign for you to motivate into action. Ignoring a problem too long leaves you open to "Rock Bottom Syndrome." Hitting rock bottom is a trigger event in which you wait for things to hit their lowest point before acting. You may be in such denial that it takes losing your job, your marriage, or something else dear to you before you wake up to the realization that you must change. While trigger events are essential for change, they do you no good if you do nothing about them.

Triggers may cause a sense of doubt, hesitancy, or confusion, but be careful not to simply move on once the event passes—as tempting as it may be. Ignoring trigger events is, itself, a negative pattern, prompting repetitive and deepening feelings of self-disgust and hopelessness. And ignoring such feelings about yourself won't make them go away. The reality is quite the contrary: Those feelings take up residence within you until you deal with them. If there is an area in your life that really needs changing, the feeling will come up again and again, triggered by a variety of causes.

A trigger event can be accompanied by the realization that your life's current course is no longer acceptable and that something has to change. Often, with a trigger, there's a realization that only you can take the action required to make change happen. Although such a realization may at first seem overwhelming and frightening, in the final analysis, it's extremely empowering when accompanied by the crucial next step of creating and implementing a plan.

It might help to think about these events (which may be painful and disappointing) as positive opportunities, and quite possibly, as the beginning of something great. Once again, while trigger events are essential, they do you no good if you take the process no further than the "Aha!" point. Sometimes in order to get off a negative course, you need a jolt—something "in your face" that forces you to look at a situation and perhaps at yourself from a whole different perspective. Trigger events are opportunities for change.

One of the more interesting cases about trigger events and change involves lawyer Christopher Darden, who came into prominence with the O.J. Simpson trial. In reading about him, I was struck by how he traveled a long way from his humble origin to such prominence. He could not have done it unless he had broken certain patterns that interfered with his vision of what he wanted, and had set goals toward achievement.

Darden grew up in a low-income, African-American community near San Francisco, where the idea of pursuing a career in law seemed distant, if not impossible. In his autobiography, *In Contempt*, he reacted against his early uncertain future by "criming and conniving. It was how I existed. Cynics might say my lawyerly character developed early . . . I stole in elementary, junior high, and high school."

He stole despite the fact that he excelled in sports and received decent, if inconsistent, grades. He reached a turning point at the end of ninth grade when he brought home a report card with three A's and three F's. Obviously, he had the intelligence to excel when he put his mind to it. Yet, he was very close to failing out. "One more F, and I'd be just another high school drop-out," he wrote. "I can't say it was an epiphany . . . I only knew that I wanted to get out of there and be whatever man I could hope to be."

He focused on his studies and on his budding desire to have a career in law. He went to college and excelled on the track team and in campus politics. Still, Darden was unable to envision his future. It seemed safer to focus on track than on books. He also continued his custom of stealing. As a pre-law criminal justice major, he'd have been expelled immediately for any arrest, yet he continued his long-ingrained habit of shoplifting food and clothing.

Darden gives credit to a history professor for bolstering his self-esteem and convincing him to concentrate on class work rather than on sports. As for his illegal activities, he abandoned them for good when he found himself "lying in a muddy field, cold and miserable, eluding the police after shoplifting at Sears and marveling at how stupid I was." A vivid and powerful trigger. By finally creating a vision and developing a goal for his future career in law, he broke his most harmful patterns. He was accepted at Hastings School of Law at the University of California, and after graduation, he received a job in the Los Angeles County District Attorney's office. Prior to the Simpson case, he had successfully prosecuted 19 murder cases.

Of course, Darden's story does not end there. The failure to convict Simpson was a very public and bitter setback for him. He accepted responsibility for the public loss. With it came a personal sense of loss, too. He lost some of the drive to be a trial lawyer and resigned his post as a prosecutor. "I couldn't go back to the courtroom expecting justice when there had been none in the strongest murder case I ever prosecuted." He rebounded from the setback by penning a best-selling memoir and donating a portion of the profits to a shelter for battered women.

Trigger Events and Conscious Insight

How can you logically find your way through a trigger event? Like everyone, you have a shot at reaching a very valuable tool in your arsenal for personal growth through a trigger event. It invariably causes you to examine your life from a new perspective. When you do, you achieve conscious insight. With *conscious insight*, you can see yourself as you really are. It's a higher level of perception than what you may be used to.

To break the pattern:

▸ Capitalize on the opportunities that trigger events offer. Don't back away, but face them head-on.

▶ Reflect on what the trigger event can mean: think about what's troubling you and holding you back. List the patterns you repeat automatically that led to the trigger event. (In the next part I'll take you through exercises that help you understand triggers and how to proceed from them.)

No Pain, No . . . Well, You Know

As humans, we are hard-wired to do whatever is necessary to avoid pain. People often face great mental and emotional resistance to looking honestly at themselves and the ways they have contributed to their own problems. But the potential rewards of doing so are immeasurable. You need to be conscious of your patterns before you can change them. Remember, patterns are self-created. And it stands to reason that whatever you create, you can also destroy. Tell yourself your own story, truthfully, in order to detect your underlying patterns. In the next chapter, there are a number of Exercises to break patterns and begin the transformation of your life.

Summing Up

- Patterns play an important part in your psychological make up, personality, and behavior. Patterns are a series of interconnected decision-making processes, the result of how your mind frames your experiences.

- Jobs and relationships travel familiar paths. If you feel like you're trapped in a never-ending circle of patterns that are getting you nowhere, you can take the first step toward recognizing the patterns you want to change and modify them. Breaking your patterns is liberating.

- One complication of not confronting problems or crises that arise from negative patterns is that you stay stuck in the past.

- Success comes from carefully examining your patterns and not placing blame on yourself or others. Instead, look for the motivation underlying your mistakes so you can correct them in the future. Holding others responsible for your failures or successes places you on the road to helplessness. You can't change other people, you can only change yourself and the way you relate and respond to people.

- Denial is equally counterproductive. Denial means you're refusing to acknowledge and act upon the warning signs that something is terribly wrong and about to cause you harm, loss, or emotional pain. If you hold onto denial, you won't be able to see, and ultimately, break a pattern.

- Don't fool yourself into thinking that life will hand you a shortcut to success, achievement, and happiness. The path of least resistance is often paved with disappointments.

- To kick-start breaking a pattern, you need motivation and a trigger event. Motivation gives you the passion to change; the trigger event gives you information as to why you should break the pattern. It can be as extreme as a humiliating personal disaster or as common as wanting to impress former friends at a reunion. With a trigger, there's a realization that only you can take the action required to make change happen.

31

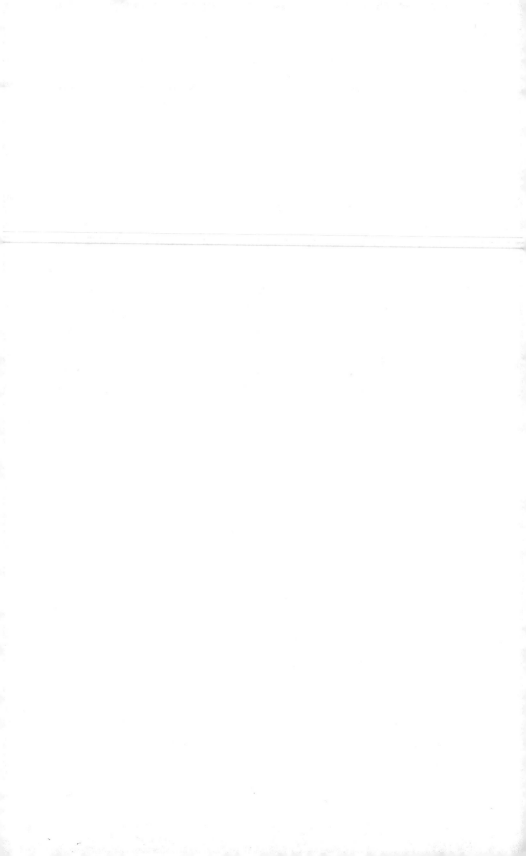

CHAPTER TWO

Self-Evaluation and Reflection Workshop— Yes, You Can Change!

God grant me the serenity to accept the things
I cannot change; the courage to change the things
I can; and the wisdom to know the difference.
—Reinhold Niebuhr

In the previous chapter, I talked about the six most common patterns of behavior that are obstacles to attaining your goals. The patterns are:

- Finding someone/something to blame
- Self-sabotage or self-paralyzing behavior
- Making bad choices compounded by denial
- Always seeking the short cut or path of least resistance
- Choosing to be overweight
- Substance abuse

The good news is that negative patterns can be broken and replaced by positive ones. The only way to change is to first want to change, and then you must do the work. In order to help recognize patterns—negative and positive, specific and general—it's essential to evaluate and reflect on your behavior. What does this mean? It means you need to watch yourself, take a look at how you are and how you act—that's how you will grow and reach your goals. Can you grow and reach your goals without self-evaluation and reflection? Of course, but it would be strictly by chance. I found that the following formula synthesizes and clarifies the importance of using these techniques:

Learning = Self-Evaluation + Reflection

While the Exercises I provide in this chapter help with the process of self-evaluation, it's up to you to reflect on the meaning of your answers and statements. I'll suggest a few techniques to aid you in reflection and honest self-evaluation. The goal is to learn about yourself without judging yourself too harshly. You must look at yourself with both a critical and forgiving eye. A harsh judgment can make you want to obscure the truth. You may have good and very valid reasons for slipping into the patterns that have characterized your life so far. But if you've gotten this far in *Breaking the Pattern*, it's because these mechanisms probably no longer serve you.

It's not unusual to camouflage certain unpleasant or unflattering details or truths about yourself—everyone does it. But an honest and uninhibited look at your history and future is a courageous and potentially healing and cathartic act. By embarking on such a voyage of self-discovery with an open heart and mind, you can expect to have an "Aha!" experience—that moment when you finally see things as they really are and identify the underlying structure that governs your behavior and personality.

Getting Started—How to Be a Detective In Your Own Life

Detectives look for patterns in crimes and criminal behavior so they can identify a "modus operandi," or method of operation. These methods or patterns of behavior are giveaways and help detectives narrow down the field of suspects to identify the culprit and, ultimately, stop the harmful behavior. All you have to do is turn on any television crime show, and you can watch the detectives (many times working with forensic experts) piece together clues to solve a mystery. This is not unlike what you need to do in your personal life. The twist in this puzzle is that you are both the sleuth and the prime suspect.

While your conscious mind attempts to uncover and eliminate negative patterns—or at least "arrest and rehabilitate" them—your unconscious mind is working to throw you off the trail. Unknowingly and unintentionally, you set booby traps to block the discovery of what causes you to repeat the patterns that get you into trouble. So if you tend to fall short of your goals, time after time, it might be because you fall into your own booby traps, time after time.

The first task for any detective is to establish the facts of the case, sometimes called a "fact pattern." In your mission to break negative patterns, you must first compile a case history, a list of what you intend to achieve and what you have actually accomplished up until now.

I first realized that this was a difficult undertaking when I received the letter from my college friend that I discussed in the Introduction. Although I was eager to write back and re-establish what had once been a valued friendship, I found myself putting off the task for many months. Whenever I sat down to write, I felt overwhelmed by the enormity of conveying 14 years of life in one letter. How could I possibly relate the triumphs and setbacks, successes and failures, and certainties and doubts in my adult life in so confined a space?

I finally sat down and gave myself a simple task: make categories of lists—important highlights of my life. I began by listing the various jobs, business ventures, and personal relationships I'd had since I'd last seen Marie. I tried to note them in chronological order, but invariably I'd forget some job/association or woman and I had to go back and insert it. I found the experience was exactly the opposite of how I'd imagined when I started out. Instead of being unpleasant, it was exciting and satisfying to see the tangible written evidence of where I'd been and what I had done.

Paradoxically, the failures and painful episodes or memories that might have been the most difficult to write about ended up being the most interesting and instructive. They were the ones that shaped me and made me grow personally. When I finally wrote to Marie, I had to choose what to tell her. I didn't want to send her an encyclopedia, and I didn't want to seem boastful, or at the other end of the spectrum, pitiful.

But the luxury of making a list for your own use is that you don't need to edit out those unflattering aspects of yourself. There is no one to fool or entertain, win over or win back. You have nothing to lose and everything to gain by being completely honest with yourself. If you have failed to achieve your goals so far, you might have trouble admitting a certain defeat to yourself. I understand how you might be afraid to confront the pain of underachieving. But you'll find that those blocks and obstacles you erect to avoid looking into sensitive areas are the ones that need the most scrutiny.

How do you begin making these revealing lists? The following exercises, which are really techniques for pattern recognition, are meant to get your mind moving and thinking. OK, now how do you open yourself up to reflective behavior and self-assessment? Here are a few ways to shake things up, and see where things land. The questions and the answers will teach you to examine the most important person in your life—you.

EXERCISE 1

Looking to Your Parents for Answers

Self-evaluation and reflection can be difficult because it's not always easy to see and assess your own patterns. I'll let you in on a little trick-of-the-trade to ease the way: If you want to hold up a mirror to examine your own negative patterns, turn the mirror just a bit to look at your parents' negative patterns. This is a great place to start.

Sometimes you realize, to your chagrin, that you're unconsciously following your parents' patterns. It's funny, but for some people (myself included), a big fear is that they'll turn into their parents. Now, I know that not everyone feels this way. In fact, I think parents get a bad rap most of the time and end up being scapegoats for all your troubles (but that's a whole other book). Beyond this, some of your parents' patterns, even the ones that drive you crazy, are actually good for you. Like it or not, there are important lessons to be learned from them. As you grow up—especially if you spend your formative years with your parents—you're not just developing your own unique positive and negative patterns, but along the way, you consciously and unconsciously adopt many patterns from your parents. Since it's easier to see negative patterns in others than in yourself, examining your *view of your parents* is a great place to start. Begin with your mother or mother-figure, whomever was more influential.

Write down five negative patterns of behavior you see in your mother or the woman who most influenced you as you grew up:

1.

2.

3.

4.

5.

Now, write down five negative patterns of behavior you see in your father or the man who most influenced you as you grew up:

1.

2.

3.

4.

5.

List the five most influential of their negative patterns that you are most likely to duplicate or have duplicated:

1.

2.

3.

4.

5.

EXERCISE 2

Looking Back

In this Exercise, examine your life and identify your choices and how you expressed yourself.

Make a list of all your personal achievements going as far back as you can remember:

1. Early years:

2. High school years:

3. College years (if you did not attend college, fill in what you did following high school):

4. Post-college years:

Make a list of your early goals, including things you wished for as a child. Next to each one of these goals (no matter how silly or uncomfortable you might feel) put an "A" next to those you've achieved and a "P" next to ones that are still pending or in progress.

Write down every job you had and state the reason you left or you were asked to leave. Be extremely specific and honest. This Exercise is not for anyone's benefit but yours.

Review the five most significant relationships you had in your life, by category.

Friends

1. Are you still in the relationship?

2. How has the relationship changed over the years, if at all?

3. What are or were the specific problems in the relationship?

4. What are or were the specific positive aspects of the relationship?

5. If the relationship ended, why? Be specific.

Boyfriends/Girlfriends

1. Are you still in the relationship?

2. How has the relationship changed over the years, if at all?

3. What are or were the specific problems in the relationship?

4. What are or were the specific positive aspects of the relationship?

5. If the relationship ended, why? Be specific.

Spouse

1. Are you still in the relationship?

2. How has the relationship changed over the years, if at all?

3. What are or were the specific problems in the relationship?

4. What are or were the specific positive aspects of the relationship?

5. If the relationship ended, why? Be specific.

Coworkers

1. Are you still in the relationship?

2. How has the relationship changed over the years, if at all?

3. What are or were the specific problems in the relationship?

4. What are or were the specific positive aspects of the relationship?

5. If the relationship ended, why? Be specific.

Now look for patterns in your personal and professional life.

1. Do your relationships usually disappoint you?

2. Do you tend to leave jobs, relationships, clients, and entrepreneurial ventures soon after taking them or do you stay too long, without getting a promotion, significant raise, or satisfaction?

3. When you don't achieve personal goals, do you tend to blame others? Blame yourself? Blame luck?

After exploring the information in this Exercise, what do you see as the problem(s), obstacle(s), or pattern(s) that, if solved (or resolved), would create a "life changing" event in your life?

Analyzing Your Answers

Now that you've honestly identified the specific issues, patterns, or problems that may be blocking your personal growth, the next step is to use the information so it can make a difference. Ask penetrating questions about what you wrote down. Michael Ray, a professor at the Stanford University School of Business, who was featured in the magazine *Fast Company*, suggests that when you ask penetrating questions, try responding to "How come?" rather than "Why?" and you'll get more useful answers. Two suggested questions are:

▸ What is it that I don't yet understand (about a particular situation)?

▸ What is it that I'm not seeing about the situation?

EXERCISE 3

Examining Trigger Events in Your Life

In Chapter 1, I discussed trigger events—those that force you to take a deep, hard look at yourself and are usually accompanied by the realization that your current life's course is no longer acceptable and something has to change. With a trigger, there's a realization that only you can take the action required to make change happen. Remember that trigger events are opportunities for change. Therefore:

Name at least three trigger events that have driven you to make a change. Be as detailed as possible about each of these events. Search for recognizable patterns, recurring events, or feelings brought on by these events. Do you resolve to lose weight and get in shape every New Year's? Is each birthday a reminder that you've postponed some long-held dream another year? Are there similarities in the ways that your relationships end?

Some examples of Trigger Events are:

▸ *Job termination*
▸ *Birthday*
▸ *Graduation*
▸ *Divorce*
▸ *Ending a relationship*
▸ *Meeting someone who changes your life*
▸ *The death of someone significant*
▸ *Retirement*

List 3 specific triggers that led you to want change:

1.

2.

3.

EXERCISE 4

Examining Your Reaction to Triggers

Use the Triggers listed above as a starting point to identify any patterns that may exist in your triggers or your reaction to these events. The purpose of this Exercise is to make you more aware of what inspires you to desire change, and more specifically, what you have been willing to do about it in the past. Here's an example:

EXAMPLE

Trigger: *Doctor said that I have am a strong candidate for Type 2 Diabetes.*

Goal: *I need to lose weight.*

Action: *I'm making a decision to start a diet on New Year's Day.*

Results: *I wanted to start my diet on January 2. I had a few friends over for the football game, and they brought over donuts, beer, bags of chips, and a bowl of dip. I ended up starting my diet on January 3rd. I stuck to it for about a week, but I didn't lose any weight. My wife baked a great lasagna, so that was that. But I'll be fine. I'll start next week.*

Using the above outline (Trigger, Goal, Action, Results), and the triggers defined in Exercise 3, write down specific instances where you encountered a trigger event that created a goal, regardless of the outcome.

1. Trigger:

    Goal:

    Action:

    Result:

2. Trigger:

    Goal:

    Action:

    Result:

3. Trigger:

    Goal:

    Action:

    Result:

Rediscovering Reflection, Great Minds, and Conscious Insight

> *There is no expedient to which man will not resort to*
> *avoid the real labor of thinking.*
> —Sir Joshua Reynolds

> *That which we do not confront in ourselves,*
> *we will meet as fate.*
> —Carl Jung

In his studies of extraordinary minds and extraordinary people, Howard Gardner, a Professor of Education at Harvard who pioneered the notion of Multiple Intelligences, wrote that the essential common feature in great achievers throughout history is their ability and habit to think deeply about themselves, not in a selfish and narcissistic way, but in such a way that brings them greater personal understanding. Such people do not live their lives on automatic pilot, but instead, tend to bring a quality of thought and awareness to even their smallest deeds and actions, parts of life that many of us take for granted or overlook. "Extraordinary individuals stand out in the extent to which they reflect—often explicitly—on the events in their lives, large as well as small," Gardner wrote in his book *Extraordinary Minds*.

Some examples:

▸ Sigmund Freud constantly thought about his aspirations and the failures that visited him along the way. His accounts of his case studies, and his analyses of his dreams served as indispensable aids in the refinement and deepening of his own ideas, and eventually, his creation of psychoanalysis. He brought the practice of introspection to a new, and much more systematic, level. Writers mine their own personal experiences for insight into larger questions. Being able to think deeply about one's self is not a technique learned in school.

▶ Virginia Woolf, who never received a formal education, is a towering figure in the literary world and a paragon of *conscious insight*. She used diaries to reflect on every aspect of her existence. Her journeys into her own mind became the basis of her influential essays and groundbreaking fiction. Her goal was anything but simple. She wanted to document what it was like to be a thinking, feeling, sentient being. She found that facing herself, even in the darkest of times, led her to new revelations.

▶ Mahatma Gandhi achieved conscious insight through walks, daily meditations, and his own invented form of reflection about the challenges of daily life. He referred to this approach as "the experiment with truth."

▶ I'll bet you never thought you'd hear Gandhi and Arnold Schwarzenegger mentioned in the same discussion, but this body builder/action star long ago realized that *conscious insight* is an essential part of any training program. "Doing an exercise movement once with awareness was worth ten times an exercise done while distracted," Schwarzenegger once said.

You may not aspire to creating a new system of thought like Freud, a new kind of literature like Woolf, or to being an international spiritual leader like Gandhi, and perhaps you'd be satisfied with a mere fraction of Schwarzenegger's wealth and muscle mass. But the point remains that in order to unlock whatever potential you have, to break your negative patterns, and to begin to achieve, you need to practice conscious insight and with it bring greater awareness and self-understanding into your daily life. Effective self-evaluation does not necessarily happen easily, and it certainly does not happen without effort. Before exploring techniques of reflection, let's discuss why so many choose not to reflect.

To see yourself from a whole new perspective, you need to challenge certain assumptions about yourself and *expand your mind* beyond your normal capabilities. The working adult world is not set up to accommodate a lot of inner and silent reflection. But sometimes, it's not the outside world preventing us from thinking deeply and effectively about our patterns and the right course of action; rather, it is our own reluctance to reflect. There's no reason to be intimidated by the notion of reflection. It's a familiar and simple process. In school, you wrote papers, answered questions, engaged in discussions, and analyzed cause and effect in order to enhance understanding and enrich your mind. In your personal life, you discuss troubling situations with your friends, spouse, and mentors.

The ancient Greek philosopher Socrates used a method of systematic doubt and questioning others to elicit a clear expression of a truth that was supposed to be implicitly known by all rational beings. This became known as the *Socratic Method*. Philosopher John Locke said that knowing is purely a thoughtful reaction to experience. Reflection is a way of questioning ourselves. To reflect and achieve *conscious insight*, you need to do more than just ask the right questions. You need time and space, which allows you to look into yourself without outside distractions.

Many people find *meditation* to be an invaluable tool for reflection, since it helps empty the mind of its usual noise. This is a continuous stream of effortless concentration that runs for an extended period of time. When meditating, remember a few basic techniques:

▸ Ask yourself a question about your life that your subconscious can work on while you're in a meditative state.

▸ Let your thoughts wander and weave wherever they like.

▸ Make sure that your breathing is even, relaxed, and natural.

Others need to just sit and think in a quiet, orderly environment. Depending on personal preferences, you might sit for a few hours in a quiet room, or listen to soothing music, and reflect. Some people experience insights while doing repetitive or "mindless" activities that stimulate the unconscious to solve problems, like jogging, showering, or mowing the lawn. These rhythmic activities that don't require the mind's full attention offer excellent opportunities to reflect. But reflection needs to start as a conscious effort; otherwise, you will lose focus.

One Reflective Technique to Consider

Julia Cameron is a successful writer, but she hasn't had a smooth road to success. She overcame a failed marriage to Martin Scorcese, and battled alcoholism. In her widely acclaimed book, *The Artist's Way*, which is a kind of primer on unleashing creativity, she describes an extremely effective reflective technique called "Morning Pages." I interviewed her and asked her to discuss this technique with me:

> People who work with Morning Pages will notice a huge shift in their consciousness and their optimism level. I almost want to call it luck, but it's probably more properly called synchronicity. The idea is to get up in the morning and write three pages by hand about anything that crosses your mind. It's strictly stream of consciousness. It's not art with a capital 'A.' It's not even really writing in the sense of setting a topic and sticking to a topic. It really is just getting up in the morning and writing, 'Boy, you know I really

hated that meeting last night in the office' or 'I forgot to call my brother back' or 'I need to buy a new vacuum cleaner.' It's all these little niggling things that you don't think have anything to do with creativity, but they are all the inner movies that we are watching, instead of being able to think more original thoughts.

Cameron thinks that most of us are usually stuck in this stream of what she calls "fretfulness, worry, anxiety, and resentment." Putting all these issues on a page can render you alert, alive, and fresh. Writing it down gets it out of your system. This allows you to take new experiences in so that you're "stocking your inner well." It's a very potent tool.

Cameron then explained further about her process of Morning Pages and how it relates to *breaking a pattern*. Doing them every day is not only a reflective technique, but it can also be used to take a pattern and break it down on a daily basis. If you have a pattern of procrastinating, the words of it would be right in your face. You would see it and think, "Oh my God, I *am* procrastinating." Being confronted with the reality of it takes all of the fun out of procrastinating. Or, you may discover you have a pattern of not speaking the truth in your relationships.

Cameron said she uses this tool on a daily basis to try and nip negative patterns in the bud. "I would say that the major negative pattern I saw and changed was being an alcoholic," she said. "Now, I'm a sober alcoholic. I drank from the time I was 19 until I was 29, and I blacked out the first time I drank. I spent ten years trying to drink like other people and I was in denial that I couldn't. Finally, I realized that competitive drinking was running me, instead. I was very much of the '60s generation, and so a lot of other issues were just swept under the rug, such as, 'Oh, we're just free.' One day, I realized, 'Drinking is not about being free. This is being a slave.' I clearly saw it and I got sober. That, to me, was a huge 'before' and 'after.'"

Here are a few of Cameron's suggestions:

▸ Try writing your own Morning Pages for about two weeks as a starting point—see how it feels.

▸ Write a letter to yourself outlining and highlighting your success and disappointments. Make the letter autobiographical.

▸ Try one of the forms of mediation reflection techniques that were mentioned—try starting with five to ten minutes per day.

EXERCISE 6
Asking the Right Questions

Questions are the most powerful tool in the reflection experience. A good question should not be easy to answer. It should make you stop for a minute. It should set off a small journey into your mind. It's best if this journey takes you on unfamiliar paths. In that way, it opens up a potentially new way of thinking and seeing things. When you think in new ways, you grow better at thinking. In this way, the mind is a kind of muscle. The more you use it, the stronger and more agile it becomes.

The questioning process is the cornerstone of inquiry. It helps to:

▸ Extend thinking skills
▸ Clarify understandings
▸ Gain feedback to learn
▸ Provide revision strategies
▸ Create links between ideas

▸ Enhance curiosity

▸ Provide challenges

Here are some questions to ask yourself to begin the process of reflection. Be very specific, and try making a list:

1. What changes do I want to make in my life?

2. What would I like to do that I am not currently doing?

3. What risks am I willing to take to achieve my goals?

4. What challenges am I willing to face?

5. Who are my role models?

6. What is standing in the way of my making the changes I need to be happier?

Analyze Your Answers

Be ready to discuss your negative patterns without being defensive. Some people do their best reflecting out loud, talking with one other person or in small groups. Too large a group dilutes the focus on whatever is troubling you and can invite the temptation to compare your life with others. Searching for similarities with others is totally beside the point. If you need to talk things out, my suggestion is one-on-one. You may find it helpful to discuss your negative patterns with people trained in human understanding, like the clergy, counselors, mentors, or therapists. Depending on your relationship with family members, you may turn to parents, your spouse, or a sibling. Sometimes you'll learn a lot about yourself and generate new ideas precisely by articulating a problem to another person.

Writing down your reflections and insights is a powerful tool. The action of writing moves the reflection from a daydream to a concrete activity, which can be the basis for decision making.

Here's the bottom line. Of any exercise or idea you can take from this Principle, none is more important than this: Whatever efforts and goals you invest in your future will be lost if you do not take the time to think about your past. You must review your behavior, review your goals, review your relationships . . . review everything! Why not spend the time focusing on the present and planning for the future, and forget the past? This is not about dwelling on the past, but instead about learning from it and moving on. As the old adage goes, "History repeats itself"—and believe me, if you don't take the time to look back now, it will.

EXERCISE 7
Going from Reflection to Self-Assessment

Self-assessment is a more formal process than internal reflection. While reflection will take you some of the distance to self-understanding, self-assessment is a more systematic, even business-like method of recognizing unconscious patterns and formulating a way out of personal ruts and frustrations. While reflection is an indispensable part of the process, you need to practice self-assessment to implement real change.

The term "self-assessment" is most often used in the business world. As an essential component of modern managerial theory, it can be applied to managing your own life as well.

Understanding Self-Assessment

The process of self-assessment can be broken down into stages to help you clarify where you are and where you are going:

Stage 1: Articulate the problem. This is where you're in a state of doubt and are perplexed by a situation.

Stage 2: Analyze the problem. When did it start? How did it develop? How does it make you feel? What effect does it have on other areas of your life? What have been the results when you've tried to correct it? Review your past behavior as though under a microscope.

Stage 3: Assign responsibility. Rather than finding someone or something to blame, get to the roots of the problem, and figure out what area to target for change.

Stage 4: Formulate and test a process or plan to overcome the problem.

Stage 5: Act!

For now, we are concerned with Stages 1 and 2 of this process. I'll discuss Stages 3, 4, and 5 in later chapters on Responsibility, Goal Planning, and Achievement. Take three or more negative patterns that you have identified and use them for Stages 1 and 2. Ask yourself the following questions for each of the negative patterns you have identified in yourself.

1. In detail, articulate the negative pattern—leaving nothing for the imagination.

2. Break down the negative pattern. How and when does it occur?

3. How and when did the pattern start?

4. What feelings does the pattern bring on?

5. What effect does your negative pattern have on others?

6. What effect does your negative pattern have on you (short- and long-term)?

7. How do you see yourself breaking or moving away from this negative pattern?

EXERCISE 8
A Closer Look at Your Life

In this Exercise, we'll concentrate on two areas of your life: "Career/Work/Professional" and "Personal." The objective is to take a detailed retrospective look at your life to explore and examine how you got to the place you are now.

Figuring Out Your Aspirations

First, let's consider a time frame. Eventually, you may want to complete a chart incorporating your whole life, but begin with a 1-year, 5-year, or even 10-year time frame. Try to reexamine the goals you set for yourself within the last 5 or 10 years. It may also help to think of life events like high school graduation, marriage, or the end of a big relationship. Such changes are often accompanied by the setting of goals, and the envisioning of a future life.

Close your eyes and picture yourself and your goals at that time. Where were you? Who were you with? How did you imagine your life? You may have to reach very deep to understand your goals. But they were always there. You must have taken whatever jobs you have taken for a reason—you had an objective like moving out of your parents' house and living on your own, paying off student loans, exploring a new industry, or building up and owning your own Fortune 500 company.

Be as specific as possible. Remember, there are no unimportant details. A goal is often the hardest to pin down, and trying to remember a past goal, is even more difficult. People have a tendency to rewrite history in their own favor—try to avoid this. If you had an objective to "make lots of money," you can write that down, but try to be more precise. How much money did you intend to make? Exact numbers are great. $50,000 per year? $100,000? Enough to just eat and survive while you worked on something else? Enough to buy a new car? A house? A block of houses?

The *Professional* column of the page includes more than strictly financial goals. Where did you intend to be at 30, 40, or 50 years old? Owning your own business? Producing a movie? Becoming a vice president of a company? Which company? Retiring from a job you didn't like and getting the pension to allow you to finally pursue your true dream? Even include details about the kind of office you envisioned yourself in, or the actor/actress you envisioned starring in your movie.

Under the heading, include the aspects of your life that do not relate to your career. Perhaps your goal is to have a meaningful and deep relationship, but maintain your own lifestyle and remain single. To get married? On the other hand, maybe your goal is to learn to be by yourself. Your goal may be to widen your circle of friends, or improve your relationship with your sister/brother. Health goals would also go under this heading. Do you want to quit smoking? Lose weight? How much weight? Perhaps you'd like to compete in an athletic event, like a marathon. Perhaps you want minor or major cosmetic surgery.

Take your time with this process; it's like compiling and visualizing a detailed wish list for your life. It could take a few hours or even a few days to think of everything. Don't censor or judge yourself. Figuring out what you want and have always wanted is a clarifying step—it will help reveal the patterns of behavior that go along with these desires, the very purpose of this Exercise.

One of the main reasons people don't get what they want in life is that they are unclear about what they want exactly. In the show "The Search for Signs of Intelligent Life in the Universe," a homeless character, played by Lily Tomlin, says very wisely, "I always knew I wanted to be someone. I see now I should have been more specific." Be specific. If you are not clear to yourself, for yourself, how can you be clear to the other people in your life?

Having laid out your *Aspirations*, now you are ready to tackle the other areas:

The Paths You've Taken

In order to reach any goal, you often must travel down many different roads to get to your destination. The objective of *Paths* explores the different roads you have traveled to get to each of your desired goals. Try to be specific and really explore the different routes you have taken. This chapter will help you to pinpoint patterns in your life.

The Steps You've Taken

Write down the *Steps* you have taken to reach each of your specific goals, regardless of whether or not they were effective. For example, if under *Professional*, you wrote the goal "Make $100,000 per year," under *Steps*, you should list which jobs you took, how long you stayed, extra work you took on the side to realize the goal, etc. Keep everything in a time frame. As closely as possible, list the dates you started and ended working at those particular job(s) or position(s).

Knowing Your Relationships

Under this heading, write everyone you interacted with at the different stages of striving toward your various goals. In the *Professional* section, this will include bosses and coworkers, or if you have been entrepreneurial, it will include partners, important clients, and backers. In the *Personal* section, list all of the relationships you've had.

Try to imagine each person's take on the event in question. Imagining another person's perspective, if it does not come naturally to you, is a difficult task, but immensely useful. For instance, if the event was the loss of a job, why do you think the boss let you go? What do you think your coworkers thought? You may disagree with these points of view, but try to explore them anyway.

A helpful step is to pick up the phone and ask these people. If you feel that you can handle it, this can be extremely useful. Don't be afraid to call an old employer, coworker, partner, or girlfriend or boyfriend and ask, point blank: "Why do you think I failed at this?" *Don't consult people who you think might want to gratuitously hurt your feelings, or those that will simply tell you what you want to hear.*

You may be surprised at the insights other people will give you. If you speak to enough people, you may suddenly become aware of some patterns you were not aware of until you heard enough people tell you about them. One person can be biased or mistaken, but if more than one person says it about you, there may be some truth to it.

Examining Outcomes

This can be a difficult section, since it forces you to confront the results of all your efforts, no matter what they were. Try to record the outcomes of your various pursuits without judgment. If you were fired from a job, say so. If you quit or left the business, say that. Be honest about how personal relationships ended. Make sure to write down the reasons why the outcome turned out the way it did. Look for patterns.

You do not need to concern yourself with why things turned out the way they did for each of these outcomes. You may already begin to see patterns just in the details of your personal case history. To deepen your understanding of what you've learned about yourself so far, I'll analyze Failure and Responsibility in two upcoming chapters.

When you're faced with obstacles in life, you have two options: change the obstacles or change yourself in order to overcome them. Make sure that you don't skip over these Exercises—they will help you and stimulate thought. Remember that, at first, it will be uncomfortable to think about yourself this way, but it will be valuable in the long run.

Now you're ready to start the Exercise. You should do this for as many specific things you can think of in each of the categories mentioned above (but try starting small with three for each). The page should start out looking like this:

Career/Work/Professional

Aspirations:

Steps:

Paths:

Relationships:

Outcomes:

Personal

Aspirations:

Steps:

Paths:

Relationships:

Outcomes:

For most people, *Aspirations* will be the broadest category.

This is a good thing. If your aspirations are not larger than your achievements, then either you didn't set challenging enough goals, or you were already astoundingly successful.

Summing Up

▶ Your conscious mind attempts to uncover and eliminate negative patterns while your unconscious mind works to throw you off the trail. Unknowingly and unintentionally, you set booby traps to block the discovery of what causes you to repeat the patterns that get you into trouble. If you tend to fall short of your goals, time after time, it's because you fall into your own booby traps, time after time.

▸ Self-evaluation and reflection is difficult because it's not always easy to see and assess your own patterns. But this can ease the way: If you want to hold up a mirror to examine your own negative patterns, turn the mirror just a bit to look at your parents' negative patterns. This is a great place to start.

▸ To see yourself from a whole new perspective, try to break certain assumptions about yourself and expand your mind beyond its normal capabilities. This means you need to do a lot of inner and silent reflection.

▸ *Questions* are the most powerful tool in a self-reflection experience—so ask yourself the tough ones. A good question shouldn't be easy to answer, but should make you stop for a minute and set you off on a small journey into your mind. It's best if this journey takes you on unfamiliar paths. In that way, it opens up a potentially new way of thinking and seeing things. When you think in new ways, you grow better at thinking, and, at breaking patterns.

▸ *Writing* down your ideas and insights is important. The action of writing moves the insight or reflection from a daydreaming state to a concrete activity that can be the basis for decision-making.

▸ Perform self-assessment and break it down into stages that help clarify where you are, and where you are going:

Stage 1: Articulate your problem with the pattern you want to break.

Stage 2: Analyze the problem. When did it start? How did it develop? How does it make you feel? What effect does it have on other areas of your life? What have been the results when you've tried to correct it?

Stage 3: Assign responsibility to yourself, get to the roots of the problem, and figure out what area to target for change.

Stage 4: Form and test a process or plan to overcome the problem.

Stage 5: Act to break that pattern!

PATTERNS

FAILURE

RESPONSIBILITY

GOALS

ACHIEVEMENT

CHAPTER THREE

Failure Is an Asset Waiting to Be Discovered

The mystery of life is not solved with success,
which is an end in itself, but in failure, in
perpetual struggle, in becoming.
—Patrick White

Those who pursue life without failure, never achieve.
Those who pursue life without examining and
reassessing failure, never achieve greatness.
—Anonymous

It is by my sorrows that I soar.
—Mahatma Gandhi

I'll go out on a limb here and suggest that you're reading this book because you're not altogether satisfied with your life at this point. If this is the case, perhaps what you learned about yourself from the Exercises on page 37 of Chapter 2 offered some instructive, if not somewhat painful, clues as to why.

These Exercises have asked you to basically lay out your life so you can examine where you came from and where you're going. In answering the questions, you may have gotten a reminder, or two, of the goals you set and abandoned or became too discouraged to pursue. So if you're feeling a sense of dissatisfaction in your professional, personal, or even spiritual life, then perhaps you were able to connect to your pattern of behavior responsible for recurring setbacks and disappointments. Or, your failures. In this chapter, I'll dig deeply into the meaning of "failure," drastically rethinking it and redefining it with a capital "F." I use the word in quotes for now because of the negative connotations the word brings up for most people. Inadequacy. Incompetence. Losing. Unluckiness. Doom. I believe I can show you a way to take the shame out of the experience, fear, or idea of failure and restore its dignity and its place on the continuum of striving. The good news is that you can learn from failure. It's not only OK to fail, but it's also all right to acknowledge your failures and forgive yourself for them.

It's my hope that you'll deepen your understanding of yourself by thinking of your individual failures as jumping-off points, markers on the road to success and the chance to grow. I'll examine numerous examples of failure from the worlds of science, politics, sports, and the arts to illustrate how intrinsic failure is to any meaningful journey. I'll talk about the Internet economy, a business arena with which I'm very familiar, one that has given failure a whole new meaning—a kind of badge of courage—now seen as an important building block on a resume. Of course, I'll touch on the impact of failure in your personal life, painful endings to marriages, romantic relationships, and friendships, which can be important in your growth as a more rounded, empathetic, and wiser human being. I'll show you how to apply the lessons learned from these examples of failure to change your patterns and the way you see things.

What is Failure?

The word "failure" scares a lot of people. To some, failure suggests a permanent state of being. Fail once, and you'll always be a failure. To others, failure is something undesirable that occurs once in a while and must be shut out from one's memory—fail and forget. And yet to others, failure is just simply the opposite of being successful. Most of all, nearly everyone is understandably reluctant to pursue thinking and dwelling on failure. But what about accepting such an event?

Paradoxically, in order achieve what you want, you need to embrace Failure with a capital "F" and, eventually, lose your fear of it. If you look at Failure more optimistically, as a temporary result or setback, as falling short of one's objective for the moment, each Failure will teach you a new way to approach your objectives. Failure becomes a necessary step on a path toward reaching a worthwhile goal. *Failure is an opportunity to learn and grow, and is an integral part of achievement, not separate from it.* Let me offer you a simple equation:

$$Trying + Failing = Learning$$

If, indeed, experience is the greatest teacher, it's only because we have the opportunity to learn from the experiences in which we have failed. The very word "experience" contains the notion of trial and error. It comes from the Latin word *experientia*, meaning trial of or proof of. "Experiment," which has the same Latin root, is the foundation of science. Experience can be described as trial and error experiments that produce learning. And what is life if not a grand experiment?

Samuel Lefrak, the innovative real-estate developer who became a multi-millionaire by figuring out how to build affordable housing after the World War II, said at the age of 81: "What do I attribute my success to? Two words: Right Decisions. I make right decisions and I have experience. How did I get experience? Two words: Wrong Decisions." That is, even Lefrak failed, but failure gave him the opportunity to succeed and achieve his goals.

Failure and making mistakes are not just characteristics of success; they are intrinsic and inevitable in any meaningful pursuit. Extraordinary people, or ordinary people who manage to accomplish a great deal in life, fail often because they can take enormous risks. What is important is how they react to any failures and setbacks. *They use each failure as an opportunity to learn, become stronger, and tackle the challenge with renewed gusto and refined thinking.*

Among Mark Twain's more famous lines is the one suggesting that quitting smoking is easy since he'd done it so many times. Most people do not quit smoking, kick a drug addiction, or lose a lot of weight on their first attempt. No matter how many setbacks or failures you experience in these areas, the important thing is to *get better at it,* to improve your efforts, learn something from the setbacks. Learning what does not work for you is as important as learning what does. The second Principle of appreciating failure begins with the understanding of one of our greatest fears.

Fear of Failure

Research has shown the following correlations to be true: *Low achievement is linked to a high fear of failure; high achievement is linked to a low fear of failure.*

To explore this link between achievement and attitude toward failure, researchers in one study offered people a choice of three types of video games to play: The first was known to be easy, the second was unknown but assumed to be difficult, and the third was known to be extremely difficult.

Who played which game? The results looked like this:

Subjects with a *high need* for achievement almost always chose the second game. They knew it would be a challenge, but figured they could meet it and prevail. They possessed both curiosity and confidence.

People with a *low need* for achievement chose either the first game or the third game. In the first game, their success was virtually guaranteed. In the third game, they knew they'd have an automatic excuse if they failed—that success was not really expected of them. They were afraid to attempt the second game where the outcome was unclear, and the chance of failure too uncomfortable a prospect.

Another study was equally revealing. In this experiment, subjects were asked to take a test twice. After the first round, they received feedback such as, "You got 82 percent correct." Then they were asked to take the test again. The results were interesting:

People with a *high need* for achievement increased their efforts by preparing for the next test, regardless of the results of the first test. They interpreted any feedback as a spur to improve their performance. Meanwhile, people with a *high fear* of failure tended to decrease their efforts. Either they had already met their goals, or they took the initial score as a discouraging sign that they couldn't do better than 82 percent and would fail to improve, so why try?

Apparently, high achieving people experience failure differently from those who do not extend themselves to achieve. While no one likes to fail, some people take it as a greater challenge, and as a result, become more determined, more thoughtful, and more creative. Failure provides a chance to problem-solve that wouldn't be available if everything had gone 100 percent smoothly. People who achieve hold onto the belief that they cannot fail in any permanent way. They will eventually meet their goal, one way or another. *While they may experience failure, they will never concede to defeat.*

On the flip side, people who fear failure and want to avoid it at all costs are reluctant to attempt anything that might lead to a dreaded outcome. They are crippled by their fear of failure, which makes them afraid to take risks or compete. Fear of failure carries with it a limited vision, and people with it cannot see any way out that doesn't involve the certainty of loss. Paralyzed into inaction, they spend their days quieting the nagging sense that they are not living up to their potential. They shorten their scope of achievement, opting to remain in a safe and comfortable zone where success—or at least what they see as success—is guaranteed.

If you feel this way, you can learn to calm your fears by knowing that any new situation comes with some uncertainty. Think back to the first time you drove a car, for example. Childhood is full of firsts, including the ups and the downs—that's part of its exhilarating experiences. In fact, it may be that you developed your aversion to risks as a result of some childhood experience associated with taking chances in a new situation, or some trauma. Wanting to recover some of that exhilaration can help propel you into more risk-taking and experimentation, without which there is no growth.

Understanding Fear

I've always regarded fear as one of the greatest inhibitors of success, one of the great oppressors of human growth. Fear of learning, fear of failure, fear of change, fear of commitment, and the list goes on and on. I try to pretend that I'm not afraid of anything, but that's just not true—I have plenty of fears which I continue to tackle "inch-by-inch" until they are gone.

Anthropologist and author Carlos Castañeda in his discussions with the mystic Indian, Don Juan, talked about "challenging your fears, until they are no more." Castañeda found this confusing, so Don Juan explained further. He said that if you continuously challenge your fears, eventually you'll have no fears left. The point is not to let your fears keep you from your dreams, and to challenge them every moment of your life.

EXERCISE 1

Recognizing Fear

Write down your 10 greatest fears:

1.
2.
3.
4.
5.
6.
7.
8.
9.
10.

What 10 things would you do differently if you had no fears?

1.
2.
3.
4.
5.
6.
7.
8.
9.
10.

Anticipation of Fear

Many times the anticipation of fear is worse than the actual pain of the situation you're worried about. Remember the cliché, "You are your own worst enemy"? Well, it's a clear fit under these circumstances. Often, you may put your fears in the direct path of your goals (a common form of self-sabotage). Recent studies focusing on the fear of pain and its relation to pain itself were very revealing. Dr. Alexander Ploghaus at Oxford University did brain scans of people who were expecting pain and "found that a certain area was activated, which may help prove a theory that the fear of pain is worse then the pain itself. One knows the situation where one clings to the dentist chair in anticipation of pain and probably because of that finds the pain subsequently gets more intense than if they relaxed," said Dr. Ploghaus in an interview with *The New York Times*.

Remember: Keep your fears in perspective, learn about them, understand them, and then overcome them.

Don't Dwell on Failures and Mistakes

Is it important to remember and understand your failures and mistakes? Absolutely. But you also need to pay attention to what works, what feels good, and what gets you into your "zone." Whenever you have a successful moment, you must notice it—not just during the moment but hold onto it after the moment—and reflect on that success. Remember: Don't dwell, but reflect. There *is* a difference.

Failure and the Divided Self

Humans are constantly evaluating themselves, which causes both pain and growth. You measure yourself against the world, against your ideal vision of what you feel you should be. You interpret yourself with the cues you receive from the outside world, starting with your parents' expectations of you. You measure yourself against reality as you perceive it and then, conversely, you measure reality against your ideals. When one falls short of the other, you experience disappointment, and wonder why things are not as you think they should be. Nevertheless, you go on measuring.

Measuring and comparing are the first things children learn to do in kindergarten. They compare how tall they are, how they draw, how neat or messy they are, and if they are "cry babies" or not. As an adult, you measure yourself, instead, against your dreams, your past, against others' expectations of you, of ideas of what you should be, even your illusions about what *could* be. Eventually, you create a scale upon which to measure yourself. You pin your self-image on this self-created scale and keep returning to it to see how you are measuring up.

Failing and succeeding are cyclical processes, each creating very different thoughts and feelings. Failure initiates a division within the self, and when the self feels divided, it sees itself as flawed and in need of repair. This produces the painful part of failure.

Failure stops you in your tracks, and will not permit you to coast along happily and without being self-conscious. The self, looking for unity again, seeks a cause, an explanation for its failure. It can only begin to heal once it takes responsibility for failure and for addressing it. By its very nature, failure opens up a route to deeper self-analysis and awareness.

A Who's Who of Failure

Everyone who achieves any sort of lasting and meaningful success has failed not once but, in many instances, hundreds of times. Inventions can take thousands of tries to get them working. Most of us, though, can look at our lives and make a list of what would be considered "failures."

Here's a resume of one man's life:

Age 22 — Failed at business

Age 23 — Ran for legislature and lost

Age 24 — Again failed in business

Age 25 — Elected to legislature

Age 26 — Girlfriend died

Age 27 — Had nervous breakdown

Age 29 — Defeated for Speaker of the House

Age 31 — Defeated for Elector

Age 34 — Defeated for Congress

Age 37 — Elected to Congress

Age 39 — Defeated for Congress

Age 46 — Defeated for Senate

Age 47 — Defeated for Vice President

Age 49 — Defeated for Senate

Age 51 — Elected President

The man, if you have not already guessed it, is Abraham Lincoln, widely regarded as the most admired and important of America's presidents. Lincoln also encountered difficulties in his early life before he entered the political arena. He lost his beloved mother when he was nine years old and his sister ten years later.

The world of politics is obviously chock-full of winners and losers. In fact, failure and defeat are a necessary part of any political career. Names that now take their place in history had to endure the very public humiliation of defeat on their way to the presidency and other high offices. Richard Nixon, Ronald Reagan, and Bill Clinton each lost important state or national elections on their way to the White House. And Richard Nixon, disgraced out of the White House, later took his place as a great elder statesman, proving that even the most infamous failure can be turned around.

There are plenty of examples in the field of athletics, too, an area in which there are obvious winners and losers in terms of skills, talents, and endurance. And no one, no matter how talented or skilled, wins all the time. Michael Jordan, the man whom many regard as the greatest and most dominant athlete in the history of sports, was cut from his high school varsity basketball team when he was a sophomore. He never stopped practicing his shots, and eventually, he made the NBA.

In his first seven seasons in pro ball, the teams Jordan played for never won the championship. These losses not only inspired him, but also taught him how champions are made. By watching how the great players on victorious opposing teams played—such as Magic Johnson and Isaiah Thomas—Jordan learned something significant: He could make the whole team better by playing unselfishly and inspiring in others the confidence he had in himself. Eventually, he led the Chicago Bulls to the championships.

Having achieved all he hoped for in basketball, Jordan became antsy and decided to try his hand at baseball. Here, the man who was deified as an athletic god became a mere mortal. As a baseball player, Jordan was not so hot, batting under .200. Recognizing that baseball was not his forte, he rejoined the Bulls and led them to even more titles.

Certainly Jordan's natural athletic ability is astounding, but it took more than that to succeed. His success came at the price of years of hard work and dedication, countless failures, and a determination to overcome defeat and improve his game.

Creative people—writers, artists, inventors, entrepreneurs, actors, choreographers—always confront the challenge of overcoming rejection and pursuing their dreams undaunted by obstacles in their paths. You might recognize some of these names:

▸ Dr. Seuss's first book, *And to Think That I Saw It On Mulberry Street,* was rejected by 23 publishers before it got into print.

▸ J.D. Salinger received more than 30 rejection notices for *Catcher in the Rye.* He kept all of them in a drawer as a reminder to continue.

- Bruce Willis, the acting superstar, stuttered throughout his youth.

- It took James Joyce many years to find a publisher for his masterwork *Ulysses*, which is now regarded by many as the greatest novel of the twentieth century.

In the pursuit of discovery and truth, scientists experiment, fail, and experiment some more as a matter of routine:

- Dr. Keeth Reemstma, chief of surgery at Columbia Presbyterian Hospital, has been trying for years to cure diabetes through transplant technology. For all his efforts and brilliance, he has failed, so far. How does he keep going? He says: "I never think of what I do as 'failure.' It's just an incomplete result. I always have in mind what I am trying to accomplish, and each experiment tells me a little more about what I have done wrong." Or, as Thomas Edison famously said after trying thousands of ways to perfect the light bulb, but still not succeeding, "I didn't fail. I just discovered another way not to invent the light bulb."

- At the age of 40, Sigmund Freud was an unknown neurologist turned-psychologist living in Vienna. After achieving prominence as a research scientist, he turned his back on that career, because something more significant happened: He became increasingly interested in understanding the reasons behind his patients' strange psychological symptoms. Then he did something no one else had done before: Listened. From listening to his patients, he developed the idea of "the talking cure." His colleagues in the scientific and medical communities considered his theories bizarre. The only people who took him seriously were other theorists who seemed like crackpots, such as Wilhelm Fleiss, who theorized that all health problems stemmed from the nose. Freud's now famous theories of the unconscious—the id, ego, and superego—did not come to him in a blinding flash. They were the result of years of clinical experimentation, study, and synthesis. Even when no one took his notions seriously, he persisted with the belief that he was on to something big. His first edition of *The Interpretations of Dreams,* a classic piece of twentieth century literature and thought, sold only a few hundred copies. However, while Freud remains controversial, he has a secure place in the Pantheon of great modern thinkers.

What do you think about failure and why do you fear it, deny it, or wish it would go away?

Let me start here:

The Power of Optimism

It's important to be honest with yourself and admit when you've fallen short of your goals. When you're able to see failure as a temporary circumstance that can be altered with improved effort, that gives rise to *an optimistic attitude, and an optimistic attitude toward life's inevitable setbacks is a cornerstone of success.*

One reason that an optimistic attitude is so important to achievement is that optimists frame their experiences so that they can learn from them. Harvard Professor Howard Gardner, who studies visionaries and extraordinary minds, describes this ability as "the capacity to construe experience in a way that is positive, in a way that allows one to draw apt lessons and, thus freshly energized, proceed with one's life." So, people who achieve great, or even modest, goals in life are not magically able to skirt failure while the rest of us struggle from obstacle to obstacle, and setback to setback. Rather, it is that optimists react to these struggles and setbacks in a wholly different way.

Martin Seligman, a psychologist at the University of Pennsylvania, has researched optimism and its relationship to athletic and academic achievement. He classifies optimists as people who see "failure" *as the result of a decision they themselves made.* Pessimists, he says, attribute "failure" to some intrinsic aspect of themselves, like having average intelligence or a limited ability with math, which they feel they cannot change—and which leaves them depressed and feeling hopeless. The difference is that optimists take responsibility for their situation and do not blame themselves for limitations or come up with an all-encompassing reason for a failure. Instead, they simply evaluate the situation and learn from it in order to make a better decision next time. Remember: Blaming yourself is just as bad as blaming someone else.

What does optimism look like in action?

Barbara Corcoran, founder of the Corcoran Group, one of the most prestigious real estate brokerage firms in New York, describes herself as someone who makes "lemonade out of lemons." Corcoran says she's "great at failure."

> This is what I've concluded. I'm great at rejection and I usually do my best in the face of failure. I've also gotten most of the creative ideas that have made money in the lap of failure, if there is such a thing. I can't say I welcome it, because each time I see it, I'm not happy to see the old guy coming back. But on the other hand, I've learned a pretty good response by now, which is, "Gee . . . something good is coming here."
>
> We're probably the leading real estate firm in the nation for Web sales. That was born out of a very bad

business idea where I opened a gallery on the Upper West Side and spent about $70,000 on the concept of creating something called "homes on tape." I videotaped all our properties, and let customers take the tapes home and view them at their leisure. This was about $70,000 more than I had, and $70,000 later, I was sitting there with 500 tapes saying, "Oh my God, what am I going to do with them?"

Then I heard of something called "the Web," and I figured I'd start a Web site and at least make some use of all this waste in tapes. In the first month, two customers bought off the site. Now, we're doing better than a sale a day, and I really believe it's the future of the real estate business. And, if not for making the mistake of putting the money into "homes on tape," we might not have our web site. We were up on the Web early and everybody said, "She's so smart to have gotten on the Web early," but all I was doing was trying to make lemonade out of lemons, so to speak.

Just as Corcoran's optimism allowed her to take risks in business, so did Olympic swimmer Matt Biondi's optimism allow him to prevail as an athlete. Biondi, the record-shattering American swimmer, had high hopes going into the 1988 Olympic Games. Some people in the sports world thought Biondi so dominated the sport that he would match Mark Spitz's 1972 record of seven gold medals.

In his first event, Biondi finished in third place. In the 100-meter butterfly, his next event, he missed the gold medal by a few hundredths of a second. Commentators speculated that these "losses" would break Biondi's spirit for the upcoming events. Far from it, they only seemed to harden his resolve. He regrouped and went on to win gold medals in his 5 remaining races.

Dr. Seligman was not surprised. He tested Biondi earlier that year to determine his level of optimism. For the experiment, he enlisted the help of Biondi's coach at a special event intended to showcase the swimmer. After the race, his coach told him his time was poor—poorer than it was in reality—and that he had to race again. After a brief rest, Biondi tried again, improving his performance, even though the first attempt had been remarkably good. So even though the coach had "lied" and deliberately underestimated his performance, Biondi was not discouraged. Meanwhile, other teammates who participated in the same study performed worse the second time around.

This sort of optimism, tempered with self-knowledge, also comes into play in academic success. In a study of 500 incoming freshman at the University of Pennsylvania, Seligman tested students for optimism and found his results better predicted their future fortunes than either high school grades or SAT scores. "What's missing in tests of ability is motivation," Seligman told *The New York Times* in an interview about the subject. "What you need to know about someone is whether they will keep going when things get frustrating. My hunch is that for a given level of intelligence, your actual achievement is a function not just of talent, but also of the capacity to stand defeated."

Seligman also studied salespeople in relation to optimism. Sales is a field in which people face rejection every day, which is why three-quarters of people going into insurance sales quit within the first three years of the job. Here, too, Seligman discovered that optimism aids success. New salespeople who were optimists by nature sold 37 percent more than those who were not. Pessimists quit at twice the rate of optimists in the first year.

The difference is clear. When a salesperson gets a "no," it is a small defeat, to be sure. A pessimist takes the defeat to heart, thinking, "I'm no good at this." Such thinking is defeatist and pessimistic because the person believes she will "never be good at this." Ultimately, she feels overwhelmed, discouraged to make any further effort, and is, in fact, rather depressed and disheartened. By contrast, rather than believing that they are forever "not good at this," optimists figure they used the wrong approach and are willing to try again.

Optimism is not a natural, or inherited trait, although it certainly helps to be raised in a family where hopefulness, persistence, and hard work are both emphasized and practiced. But even if that is not the case, optimism can be learned. I found a few critical pointers on this in Martin Seligman's book, *Learned Optimism*. They are:

▸ Changing Your Reaction to Failure:
When you fail at something or fall short of a goal, examine your reaction to the circumstances. Instead of castigating yourself or blaming someone else, outside influences, your parents, or that really mean teacher you had in junior high school, try asking yourself, "What didn't work about my approach?" or "How could I do things differently and more effectively?"

▸ Getting Real:
To be an optimist, you must use your optimism wisely. Optimism is not about existing in some dreamy, passive state in which you believe things will all work out in the end without making an effort. Instead, to use optimism realistically, hold fast to the belief that if you rethink your approach, you can do better.

▸ Faking It:
If you're inclined to feel a certain amount of pessimism and are easily discouraged, there's still good news for you. Seligman's research indicates that if you just behave as an optimist would, you

reap the benefits of optimism. Act optimistically, and things may very well go your way. And, who knows? Once you start behaving like an optimist and view your failures as opportunities to learn, grow, refine your thinking and your approach, you just might become one. To help you figure out your optimism levels, try the following Exercise:

EXERCISE 2

How Optimistic Are You?

Return to the Exercises you did in Chapter 2 (page 38). Select one of your aspirations that has not been fulfilled, perhaps even one that you have given up on. Think about why you put it aside. Do you hear yourself saying things like: "I'm not really good at . . ." or "I'm not smart enough to . . ." or "People like me never get . . ."

Examine the routes and methods you used to try to reach that goal. Did you start out feeling sure of yourself, or sure of the idea and hopeful things would work out? When did you start feeling your optimism and confidence eroding? When did you hit the wall and stop? What or who stopped you? Is there a way that you could have approached the problem differently? Be specific in analyzing the steps and where you might have gone off-course.

Finding Dignity in Failure

People fail because they have plans and goals and invest
themselves in projects to attain their goals.
If people did not do things, to try and act upon their worlds,
if they did not propose to actualize inner wishes and dreams,
there could be no sense of inadequacy, misfortune or error . . .

It is from the idea that we should succeed that failure is born.
—David Payne, author of *Coping with Failure*

*For me, there are two kinds of failure: Succeeding
at something you hate, and failing at something
you love. I have, at various times, done both.*
—Jerry Stahl, sitcom writer and novelist

There is a dignity in striving, in trying your best, even if it falls short of your goal. In certain kinds of competition, like sports and politics, it is a simple fact that not everyone can win. The satisfaction and dignity comes from having done one's best. More often than not, when you take a clear look at a situation, define your reason for failure, then plan bold and decisive action, you will prevail; if not with your first efforts, then over time, if you stay at it. Often, reaching goals is a matter of stamina and patience.

Here's an example of perserverence in the face of adversity regarding Maury Povich, the television talk-show host. Journalism runs in Povich's family. His father was the sports editor of the *Washington Post.* His sister was a senior editor at *Newsweek.* He even married into the business—his wife is Connie Chung, a nationally known newscaster. Although he currently hosts his own daytime television show, Povich's path was anything but smooth. He admits that he distinguished himself at a young age by being mischievous. "I was sort of my father's bad boy," he said.

He went to the University of Pennsylvania after high school, but was kicked out for poor grades. His father set him straight and he finally graduated at age 23. Soon he was working as the host of "Panorama," a popular daytime talk-show in Washington, D.C. After a few years, he was bored and restless. The NBC affiliate in Chicago hired him, but this move turned out to be a disappointment, as Povich did little more than battle the station management over his contract. Soon after, he moved to CBS in Los Angeles, where he and Connie Chung anchored a newscast together. Then Povich was fired for low ratings. "I was shattered to the core," he later told *People* magazine. "I began wondering if I should be selling shoes." His marriage (not to Chung) ended at about the same time. For a while, his career was anything but stable. He moved to San Francisco, then Philadelphia, then back where he started, to Washington, D.C. Despite the adversity, he persisted in a business that loves winners and is cruel to those on the outside.

His fortunes turned when media mogul Rupert Murdoch offered Povich the host spot on "A Current Affair," a new tabloid television news show. Povich's trademark smirk and quick wit were responsible in large part for the show's popularity. He made the audience feel like he was one of them. He then used that winning ability to launch his own daytime talk-show. Povich described his route to success as akin to: "when you go into a deli and it's crowded and you take a number. If you hang around long enough, they gotta call it."

In a way, Povich was being too modest. Sticking with a career through all its ups and downs is more challenging than waiting for your number to be called. Memory may have edited out the number of times when he'd been tempted to quit the business altogether. Even when the outlook was grim, Povich stayed with the television business, sowing seeds that eventually grew into a fulfilling career. Underneath it all, he maintained a fundamental faith and optimism that with the right kind of effort on his part, "his number would be called."

Many Times Failure Is Success

Often failure is more than just an opportunity to learn and improve yourself—sometimes failure is even better than success. Success will rarely test you or make you contemplate your behavior. You celebrate it, roll along with it, and roll around in it. It feels pretty comfortable and pleasant and you hope it will last forever. It's a superficial experience, one that doesn't make you dig too deep, or think too hard, or re-evaluate, because after all, whatever you did worked, didn't it? So why not leave it alone?

Keep in mind that too much success, and not enough failure, can be problematic. It can lead to stagnation, weakness, and a lack of clear thinking.

There is a part of the human spirit that wants to be challenged and yearns to know the pride in oneself that comes from meeting a difficult challenge head-on and overcoming it through grueling thought and effort. This is achievement. Again, success can be the result of luck. *Achievement never is.*

There is something to be said about the trials and rewards of adversity. In the previously mentioned interview I did with writer Julia Cameron, she said:

> I owe a huge debt to adversity. When I was in my 20s, every-
> thing I touched turned to gold. When I was 22, I started
> publishing my work. When I was 24 or so, I was written up
> in *Time* magazine for having scooped The *Washington
> Post* on the Watergate story in the piece that appeared in
> *Rolling Stone.* My first screenwriting experience was *Taxi
> Driver.* I got married; I got pregnant. I was near the top in
> Hollywood. Then I turned 29, I lost my marriage, drank
> too much, got sober, and I would say, for a decade, was
> thoroughly frustrated as an artist. I was writing probably
> better than I had ever written. I was selling screenplays but
> the movies were not being made. By the end of my 30s, I
> wrote and directed a film, and got slammed by the critics.

Out of all this pain, public humiliation, and frustration, Cameron was able to distill the lessons she'd learned. It became her book, *The Artist's*

Way. She said of it: "I would say that if I just kept winning through my 30s, I'd never have had to learn how to stay unblocked through pain and criticism, how to stay functional through discouragement, how to turn failure into a new direction, or how to have compassion for other people. Everything would have just been about me and my brilliant career."

Cameron feels she owes a huge debt to adversity. "Failure and adversity have given me tools that success never did."

Cameron says that adversity made her a better person and a much stronger artist. It also taught her the following:

▸ Any creative career is very much like an athletic career—in any sustained athletic career, you are bound to suffer injury.

▸ People really need to develop a tool kit of coping skills.

▸ People have to think of themselves as an ecosystem that has to be maintained in a healthy way. If you're going to take out of the pond to make art, then you have to replenish the pond. If the pond gets too toxic from poisonous criticism, then you have to learn how to filter it again.

Breaking the Failure Taboo

In the business world, perhaps more than any other place, "failure" has long been a taboo subject. But that is changing. An article in *The Wall Street Journal* argued persuasively that "Failure is clearly not getting the attention it deserves . . . There has long been a nearly paranoid aversion to admitting to, discussing, or teaching about failure . . . Only in the modern age, with its focus on human action has failure become such a crushing disgrace. The good news is that companies can and do ignore distorting passions and escape with grace—even profit. When they don't, it's still worth remembering that failure has much to teach, not only to those who failed, but to others." This article was written less than a year before the 1987 stock-market crash, which dragged the U.S. economy down into a painful recession. Failure and its lessons were everywhere.

In the wake of the Internet economy fallout in 2000, failure returned to the limelight. Some of the best business schools in the country began to teach about failure and the lessons that can be learned from it. David Berg, a management professor at Yale University, was one of the first to directly address failure in the core curriculum of a major university. One of his methods is to engage students in a frank discussion of failure in their own working lives. The students hate the word, he has noticed; someone always asks if "error" or "mistake" can be used instead. He won't allow it. He uses their reluctance, anxiety, and denial to illustrate his point about how people miss the opportunity to learn from their failures because of the strong emotions surrounding it.

Management guru and author of *In Search of Excellence* and *In Pursuit of Wow*, Tom Peters agrees that failure is still a taboo subject among the business world's old guard. "There's still a prevailing frontier optimism. So we don't talk about failure, we don't write about it, we don't even think about it." But many of the young lions of Silicon Valley are changing that perspective. Kevin Compton, a general partner with venture capitalist firm Kleiner, Perkins, Caufield & Byers recently noted: "Gen Xers follow a pattern. They graduate, start a company, fail and take a job at an established firm, all the while preparing for another start-up. These kids wear their failure as badges of courage."

Indeed, this emerging attitude toward failure in business creates a valuable framework for evaluating your experiences, by pointing out the necessity of trial and error, and re-assessing the value and significance of the stumbling blocks you encounter on the path to achievement.

Where do you begin this reassessment?

Coping With and Taking on Failure in the Workplace—Part 1

Soichiro Honda, the founder of the Honda Motor Corporation said, "Success is 99 percent failure." I agree. Failure, not ambition, talent, or connections is essential to the learning curve of the most successful men and women in American business. A recent study of 191 top executives at six Fortune 500 companies found that virtually all had suffered "hardship experiences" from missed promotions, firings, and business failures. The survey, done by the Center for Creative Leadership, a research firm in Greensboro, N.C., found that executives who managed to bounce back admitted to and coped with failures. "The ability to handle failure can make or break a climb to the top," Morgan W. McCall, a research scientist for the Center, told *The Wall Street Journal.* Indeed, these setbacks often serve as trigger events for an individual to advance her career by strengthening her purpose to strive and succeed.

Throughout the history of commerce, the most successful people and the most successful businesses have been the ones who weren't afraid to admit to loss and risk failure. Ford had its Edsel. Coca-Cola unveiled New Coke, then said, "Never mind." At one point, Johnson & Johnson introduced colored plaster casts for children—a disaster for hospitals and home laundries.

Another example of corporate success in the wake of failure can be seen in the history of Intel Corporation, the world leader in computer microprocessing technology. Intel has certainly had its share of setbacks and missteps along the way. Former Intel CEO Andrew Grove has even gone so far as to say that it is better to make a wrong decision than to avoid making a mistake by hedging your bets. Putting this theory into practice, the first version of Intel's famous Pentium Processor, when released with much fanfare in 1989, was found to have a bug. Grove compounded the problem by dismissing the bug as a tiny flaw that would not affect most computers. After much criticism, he agreed that Intel would replace the Pentium Processor at no charge. When it comes to admitting failure, one can say that it's sometimes better late than never.

When Grove sought to expand the corporation, he focused more on his managerial style to see how effective he was. To effect change in this regard, he implemented intense analysis of past performances to flush out and recognize negative patterns. "Analyzing success is not truly necessary," he said in *Forbes* magazine's *Great Minds of Business.* "Success has many, many fathers and success gets told many, many times. There is, however, a tendency to walk away from failure and leave it buried. There's an enormous amount of institutional learning that gets lost because failures don't get analyzed. So the real learning is, in actual fact, what is learned from failure."

Tabuchi agrees. Nomura Securities enjoyed decades of unprecedented success as one of the world's most profitable financial institutions. However, Tabuchi actually considers the fact that the company went so long without failing a weakness. "Past success can be as much a trap as a guide," he told the *Harvard Business Review* in 1992. Rest assured, Tabuchi got his wish: in the late 90s the company suffered huge losses at the hand of the downturn in the Asian economy, as well as a pricey racketeering scandal. But true to form, Nomura shifted strategies, and was reported to have doubled their profits from 1999 to 2000—thereby demonstrating the company's resilience and ability to learn from failure.

F. Scott Fitzgerald said that in America, there are no second acts. However poetic, that idea has pretty much been debunked. He obviously did not know about and could never have imagined Steve Jobs, one of the whiz-kid founders of Apple Computer and the man behind one of the most successful products of all time, the Macintosh computer. It's well known that Steve Jobs, along with business rival Bill Gates, changed the face of world technology. But after staggering initial success in the personal computer business of the 80s, something went terribly wrong with Jobs' management style and Apple. Some blamed Apple's declining fortunes on Jobs' abrasive and megalomaniac personality.

In a *Fortune* magazine interview, he said:

> One of my role models is Bob Dylan. I learned the lyrics to all his songs and watched him never stand still. If you look at the artists, if they are really good, it always occurs to them at some point that they can do this one thing for the rest of their lives and be really successful to the outside world, but not really be successful to themselves. That's the moment that an artist really decides who he or she is. If they keep risking failure, they're still artists. Dylan and Picasso were always risking failure. This Apple thing is that for me.
>
> I don't want to fail, of course . . . I decided that I didn't really care, because this is what I want to do. If I try my best and fail, well, I tried my best.

Eventually, Jobs left the company that had been his brainchild. In the subsequent years, Apple lost market share, and was in a death spiral, having lost more than $1 billion. Sales and market shares were plummeting. Expenses were inflated. Talented people were jumping ship, and those who stayed were in denial and busy indulging in internecine battles within the company.

At this point, Jobs was asked back as interim CEO. During his first year back at the controls, the wiser 43-year-old Jobs oversaw production of the iMAC personal computer, which was hugely successful. He overhauled Apple's product line, refocusing it on what had always been the company's strength: personal and professional computers. He also restructured its personnel, manufacturing, distribution, and marketing systems. He forged an alliance with Apple's rival, the software giant Microsoft, which led to a $150 million investment by Microsoft and the promise to launch new applications for the

Mac as often as new versions of Microsoft Office for Windows. He rehired Lee Chow, the advertising genius who had helped define the original Apple campaign. The two of them created the "Think Different" campaign, which linked creative geniuses Miles Davis, Albert Einstein, and John Lennon to Apple, and set off an enormous amount of buzz about the company. The first year Jobs was back, the company pulled in $109 million in profit.

At the time he rejoined the company, Jobs owned none of its stock, and earned a salary of only $1 per year, just so his family could be on the company's health plan. He had enough money and loved the work he was doing. Additionally, there were intrinsic rewards of overcoming failure in an arena where success is anything but guaranteed. Today, the company continues to grow, and Apple stock has staged a remarkable comeback.

Another instructive story from the annals of business history concerns the rise of the retail giant Home Depot. Twenty years ago, Home Depot did not exist; the do-it-yourself home improvement business was dominated by large regional chains like Grossman's in New England, Wickes Lumber in the West, and Lowe's in the Southeast. Of those three, only Lowe's has survived the Home Depot blitzkrieg.

According to *Forbes* magazine, Lowe's watched sales fall 30 percent from 1988 to 1995. As Home Depot began surpassing Lowe's as the top do-it-yourself retailer, Lowe's management realized they had failed to understand shifting customer needs. To get a better handle on what customers wanted, they commissioned an exit survey of 2,400 customers. The survey showed that Lowe's smallish 20,000 square foot stores and personalized service were not what customers wanted.

Lowe's then moved quickly and decisively. The company began converting its stores en masse to five times the space, the 100,000 square-foot size. It even hired a senior Home Depot executive and freely copied the strategies of its more successful competitor.

Lowe's also implemented a secondary strategy of supplementing its inventory with a variety of home appliances. Lowe's designed their stores to be brighter and more appealing to female shoppers than Home Depot's, since their surveys indicated that women were more often than not the initiators of home-improvement projects.

Sales have steadily risen since Lowe's made these changes, making it the only one of Home Depot's competitors to survive and thrive under the onslaught.

Tactics and Strategies for Turning Failure into an Asset

What Lowe's did is instructive for business but also for anyone facing the challenge of failure in any area of life. Let's look again at their strategies:

1. **They faced failure**. Sometimes we want to avoid facing the fact that what ever strategy we've adopted is not working. The sooner we face up to failure, the sooner we can do something about it.

2. **They analyzed the causes**. Since they were not sure what they were doing wrong, Lowe's consulted their customers for a fresh perspective on the market. Sometimes, our lives are too close to us and we can't see what we're doing wrong. This is why the exercises and techniques of reflection—writing things down and talking things out described in the previous chapter are useful. Sometimes, just as Lowe's did, it's smart to consult outside sources for insight into what's going wrong. It is also important to choose the right people for that task.

3. **They took responsibility**. Lowe's swallowed their pride and acknowledged that they had failed to detect the shift in their customers' shopping patterns. To get out of the rut of a bad pattern and, ultimately, failure, we need to swallow pride and admit we

need help and advice. Then, like Lowe's, we can rededicate ourselves to fixing the problem.

4. **They set goals/created a viable model**. Copying a successful model can be a good start. If there is someone in your life who is achieving what you hope to achieve, *figure out what they did to get there, and freely copy some of their techniques*. You don't have to reinvent the wheel every time. As Picasso said, "Good artists create, great artists steal."

5. **They innovated**. Don't be a slave to a pre-existing program. You may have insights into the situation that no one else does, so trust your creative instincts and innovate. Lowe's used their idea for adding appliances to appeal more to women shoppers, an innovation that worked.

6. **They took action**. Once they realized what needed to be done, Lowe's wasted no time in rebuilding their stores. They were quick, decisive, and proactive. If you don't act, it doesn't matter whether or not you had the best ideas about how to handle your problem.

Failure and Rejection in Your Personal Life

Many moving songs, poems, and stories attest to the fact that romantic rejection, that is, failure, is among life's most painful experiences. The novelist and Vietnam veteran Tim O'Brien compared the trauma of heartbreak to the trauma of war. Many people are so ashamed of having loved and lost that they have trouble admitting it, trying to convince themselves and others that there was a mutual parting of the ways, with one no more battle torn than the other. The self tries desperately to protect itself from such injurious rejection, that cuts to the core.

This may surprise you, but there is a distinct upside to this sort of wound to the ego. Rejection and heartbreak pretty much blow you open and force you to summon resources, both internal and external, to understand why you're in pain, and why your efforts have not led to your intended results. Being hurt opens up new pathways to the self, to a deeper knowledge of your motivations and desires. It teaches you lessons, as all failures do, about how to better go about things in the future, including how to make smarter choices in choosing a mate. If you jump right into a new relationship to make yourself feel better, and avoid thinking clearly, you soon realize you're repeating history and have done yourself a disservice.

Being in a developed personal relationship produces vulnerability that can lead to failure and rejection. In this busy world everything is moving at increasing speed—communication, information, transactions of every sort. So, if failure and rejection make you stop and really think deeply about yourself, and the ways in which you try to reach goals and attain satisfaction—it's not all bad.

The Critical Point

When you realize you have failed at something, you will probably reach a critical point, that determines how the rest of the story will go. Will the failure make you bitter, hard, and permanently discouraged? Will you want to just give up on the dream immediately? Maybe you think you should just resign yourself to being alone, or being poor, or being second best, or being fat? It is too painful to keep trying and to risk failing again. Or is it?

There is the other route: the optimistic route. This is also the realistic and therapeutic route that helps you seek understanding of what went wrong so you can change. You can track the error and figure out how to correct it next time. It's painful to fail, but it's even more uncomfortable to just give up. Instead, grant yourself the gift of perseverance.

Remember: Pieces of your true self are revealed in crisis—and what is a failure but a crisis of the self that has bumped up against a dream? Keep in mind that your true self and your dreams are at stake—the very essence of your being—and *how you react to crises determines everything.*

How to Get Out of the Failure Maze

As Henry Ford said, "Failure is an opportunity to begin again more intelligently." If the introduction of this Principle has done its job by taking some of the sting out of the word "failure," then you should feel better prepared to examine it in your life. I'm going to ask you to acknowledge it, not mince words about it or try to protect your feelings—in fact, I believe that deep down, most people know when they've failed. For now, do not console yourself by saying, "I tried my best and fell short." This can be just as self-defeating, since there is always room for improvement. Chances are, you can try to do better and act smarter.

EXERCISE 3

Charting Failure

Let's create a chart of your Failure history. Don't think of this as a résumé of failures—that would sound too daunting and discouraging. Think of it as a list of experiences from which you have learned. This chart represents what you have learned and what you can use in the future.

1. In the chart on page 98, list 3 situations in which you did not reach your intended goal or outcome.

    Put your failure to meet goals in specific terms. For example, if your goal was to make $100,000 this year and you made only $50,000, list the exact numbers rather than just saying, "I failed to make the money I wanted." If you wanted to be thin by the end of the year, and you actually gained weight, say so. Don't ignore the numbers and avoid getting on the scale: Write down your target weight and your real weight.

For things that don't have exact numbers, try to be as precise as possible. For example, if a personal goal was to control your temper, try to remember exact instances when you lost control. Where did such events take place, who was present, and so on?

Don't be afraid to face failure or mistakes head-on.

2. Focus on why it didn't work out.

Now that you have noted the instances in which you didn't meet certain goals or intended outcomes, let's focus on why it didn't work out.

Return to the chart on page 98 and fill in the column titled "Why I Didn't Reach My Goals."

In this area, make sure you look at your gut reaction in each situation. If you failed to advance your career or to make a certain amount of money, write down why you think that happened. Maybe your gut reaction is that your boss had something against you. Maybe you thought you were in the wrong business. Perhaps you think you just had plain bad luck. If you are a pessimist, you might think the failure resulted from a deep and unchangeable character flaw. When dealing with your personal life, write down your first thoughts of why a relationship didn't work out, or why you didn't meet some weight loss or fitness goal.

3. Examine these gut reactions and look for patterns.

   Fill in the third column on page 98 titled "Looking for Patterns." As you fill in this column, ask yourself the following questions:

   ▸ Do you tend to set unreasonable goals, or set unreasonable time limits that make it more likely that you will fail and disappoint yourself?

   ▸ Do you set yourself up for failure?

   ▸ Do you tend to blame other people or forces beyond your control?

   ▸ Do you tend to blame some inherent characteristic deep within yourself?

   ▸ How do you react to failure? Are you easily discouraged?

   If you can see clearly that your approach might have been wrong but now you can tackle the same goals using a different approach, then you may be on the right track.

4. Figure out what you've learned.

   Fill in the column on Page 98 titled "What I've Learned." This is the most critical component of this process—analyzing your experiences to facilitate learning. As you examine your experiences, look both internally and externally—consider how you behaved, as well as the individuals and/or circumstances you chose to involve in this process.

FAILURE TO REACH YOUR GOAL OR INTENDED OUTCOME	WHY I DIDN'T REACH MY GOALS	LOOKING FOR PATTERNS	WHAT I'VE LEARNED

EXERCISE 4
Looking Back in Order to Look Forward

Chances are, the course of your life has not turned because of one event, like the results of a test or the outcome of a relationship. In this section, it may be tempting to feel regret, feel sorry for yourself, or romanticize your past, making it more fulfilling than the present. Some people who were shining stars in high school may feel a nagging disappointment about what their lives have become.

Regret, however natural, is a big waste of time. Why should you concern yourself with something that's in your past, that you can't change? It is significantly more fruitful to use the lessons of the past to fashion a better future for yourself than to dwell on what "could have been." This Exercise will help you drill down to learn from past failures. Remember that the purpose of this or any of these Exercises is not to beat yourself up all over again for some past failure. By cataloging what you've learned from past failures, mistakes, and experiences, you can truly move forward unhindered by regret. Start here:

The five biggest mistakes I ever made were. (Don't skip anything—include all the details!)

   1.

   2.

   3.

   4.

   5.

The mistakes I often repeat are:

What impact does the fear of failing have on my relationships?

What impact does the fear of making mistakes or failing have on my work life?

What impact does the fear of making mistakes or failure have on my dreams?

My upbringing taught me that making mistakes or failing is:

EXERCISE 5

Moving Beyond the Fear of Failure or Making Mistakes

After taking the emotional "sting" out of mistakes and failure, re-evaluating past experiences as learning exercises, and learning from the lessons through your experiences, the next step is to search for the scars these experiences may have left behind.

These scars may reveal themselves as a fear of failure or mistakes, and unassertiveness in your strategies to achieve your life's goals. As you work through these Exercises, keep in mind your newfound perspective on past failures and mistakes that have shaped your experience.

Answer these questions:

List 10 lessons you have learned "The Hard Way."

   1.

   2.

   3.

   4.

   5.

   6.

   7.

   8.

   9.

  10.

List five things that you would never even think of doing that coworkers, family members, and friends have done to reach their goals.

   1.

   2.

   3.

   4.

   5.

List 10 situations that you fear most.

   1.

   2.

   3.

   4.

   5.

   6.

   7.

   8.

   9.

  10.

What is your greatest fear . . .

. . . in business or your career?

. . . in your personal life (i.e., relationships)?

At a job interview or business meeting, you often fear the following:

When you go on a date or start a new friendship with someone, you often fear the following:

Moving Beyond Failure

I want to reiterate the following points about Failure, with a capital "F," as you make your way through *Breaking the Pattern*. I know you will be able to glean something wonderful from your experiences—something you can learn and use. Never think that the purpose of going back over the details of your life is counterproductive. I've created these exercises so you can move forward, by looking back.

Remember, I'm not suggesting that failure and rejection are so instructive that you should actively or carelessly pursue either of them. Failure and rejection are bound to visit anyone who strives for prizes in life and is not satisfied with the status quo.

Summing Up

▸ Failure is not the opposite of success. Everyone who achieves any sort of lasting and meaningful success has failed not once, but many times, even hundreds of times.

▸ Paradoxically, if you embrace failure rather than avoid it, you can eventually lose your fear of it.

▸ When you think of failure in more realistic terms—that is, as a temporary result or setback or falling short of your objective for the moment—you can't help but succeed.

▸ When you're able to see failure as a temporary circumstance that can be altered with improved effort, you feel more optimistic. An optimistic attitude is important because it allows you to *frame your "failed" experiences so you can learn from them.*

▸ The most successful people and the most successful businesses are the ones who aren't afraid to admit to loss and risk failure. Taking that risk is a key ingredient to eventual success.

▸ To face the challenge of failure in any area of your life, you need to follow these six steps:

1. Face failure.
2. Analyze the causes.
3. Take responsibility.
4. Set goals.
5. Be innovative.
6. Take action.

▸ To break your patterns, get out of a rut, and ultimately, work through failure—take the leap—swallow your pride and admit you may need help and advice.

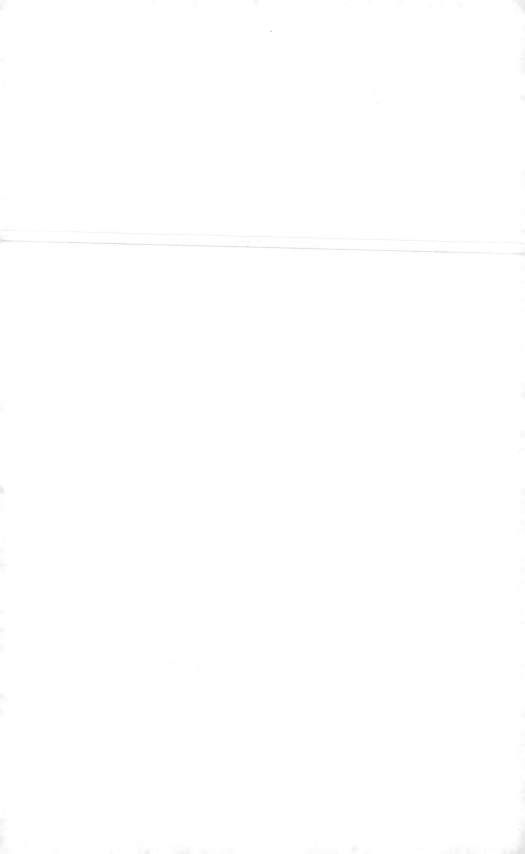

PATTERNS

FAILURE

RESPONSIBILITY

GOALS

ACHIEVEMENT

CHAPTER FOUR

Taking Responsibility Leads to Freedom

The price of greatness is responsibility.
—Winston Churchill

Although we can't always avoid the storms in our lives,
we can control our response; we can trim the sails,
batten down the hatches and make the best of it.
—Dan Millman, former Olympic Gymnast

My wife and I were out biking one Saturday afternoon along the streets of Manhattan with cars weaving in and around us. Since it was quite dangerous, I was a bit worried about my wife. She's not from New York and is a lot more trusting of local drivers in heavy traffic areas. As we were going through a green light, I thought I lost her. Momentarily caught off guard, I stopped short in the middle of the street and was thrown over the handlebars of my bike. A crowd gathered, and someone offered to call an ambulance. I was only slightly injured, but I was embarrassed, then angry.

Who could I blame?

Well, it really *was* my wife's fault—wasn't it? I mean, if I hadn't been concerned about her welfare, and if she had kept up with me, then I wouldn't have stopped short! Wow! Why not blame her?

While it's clear that this minor accident was nobody's fault but my own, it's a classic example of how easy it is to avoid taking responsibility. I'm the only one responsible for my actions. I made a choice to be concerned for my wife's well-being and my being pitched over the handlebars had nothing to do with her.

Taking responsibility.

I know it sounds puzzling and familiar at the same time, yet it's a concept that's frequently forgotten or abused during the course of our lives. What the heck does it mean? It's simply this: Control over your life doesn't arise from dodging and avoiding difficulties, but instead from coping with the issues (minor and major) that come your way or that you create. Personal honesty, conflict, and struggle constantly force you to make decisions concerning who you are as a person, and these choices are powerful growing tools. The best way to prepare for them is to *stay aware of your actions.* Only then can you become more responsible—and the payoff is a more effective life. Responsibility is choice, free choice. It means being able to determine your destiny.

This Principle promises to change your notion of what it is to take responsibility for yourself. It will help you recognize and identify responsibility-avoiding behaviors and patterns in both your professional and personal life.

Defining Responsibility

Responsibility has gotten a bad rap. Too many of us associate it with punishment and blame, both negatives. Or you may associate responsibility with dreary lectures detailing your duties and see it solely as a burden. There is a moral dimension to responsibility, but that is only part of it. Think about the word. It contains the word "respond" and the word "ability." Responsibility is, therefore, the ability to respond. An event occurs, a relationship or business fails. You suffer a loss or a setback. How do you respond? Can you get over it? Can you get past it? Can you keep heart and soul together and remain compassionate? To respond ably, or to respond responsibly, you figure out what went wrong, and determine how you can fix it, and even incorporate the setback into a well-thought out plan of action.

You may not be fully responsible for every event in your life. Accidents do happen, both lucky and unlucky ones. But you are solely responsible for how you respond to those events, and how you allow those events to shape you. Many of your own patterns, which you are in control of, not luck or chance, bring you opportunity, success, and failure.

There are very specific ways you think of yourself and how you act and react, and for the purpose of clarification I've organized them into eight general "types" of people. Each "type" has its peculiar syntax, behavior, and stock phrases. By examining these types and how they experience themselves, you can probably find a description (in part or in whole) of where you fit in. The types are:

- ▸ The Blamer
- ▸ The Higher Authority
- ▸ The Victim
- ▸ The Excuse Maker
- ▸ The Avoider
- ▸ The Counter Puncher
- ▸ The Ingratiator
- ▸ The Martyr

The Blamer

Here's Rita, a woman who is considering her day at work in a string of thoughts. "My boss rejected my marketing plan again. What else is new? Tom doesn't take my ideas seriously. He's incompetent . . . The people I work with are such losers, no wonder I go home tired and depressed. They're bringing the whole department down . . . They're all talk and no action . . . I don't know why I stay at this company . . . I'm so much better than this. The project failed because my employees are lazy. . . . They don't know the meaning of hard work . . . They've always been this way."

Caught up in the momentum of her thoughts about what's going wrong around her, she jumps to the problems in her relationship. She thinks about her boyfriend . . . "Bob is the reason this relationship is terrible . . . He cheats on me all the time . . . Bob's always been a cheater . . . Now that I think of it, when I met him he was dating someone else."

What's happening with Rita?

When something you're involved in or working on seems to be stalled, disappointing, has poor results, or ultimately falls apart or implodes, you can have one of two responses: you either *externalize* or *internalize.* Which response you favor will depend on what sort of person you are. Let me add a warning note here: You can behave differently under different circumstances; therefore, you can be an externalizer in one situation and an internalizer in another.

When you *externalize,* you look outside yourself for the reason something has happened. If you're disappointed or angry, it's because you think other people "have not pulled their weight" or "lived up to their end of the bargain." Rita believes this.

Sometimes, we scapegoat one particular person. In a business setting, that person usually gets fired. An alcoholic may also look to blame someone other than himself, saying for instance, "My spouse is so critical and demanding, she makes me drink." When a relationship fails, externalizers can attribute all the problems to the other person, often ignoring destructive patterns and behavior that seriously got in the way of its success. Or, some may blame an entire gender for not having a good and lasting relationship. ("You can never please any woman. She just takes." Or, "Men are selfish and never grow up.") Criminals are notorious for blaming "society" and any and every source outside themselves for their criminal behavior.

In all these cases, an externalizer uses a short-term strategy: to get himself or herself off the hook. As an externalizer, if your only aspiration is to remain "off the hook" (or out of jail in the case of the criminal) then this strategy just might suffice. If you're reading this book, I suspect you have higher aspirations than this. Remember, by not being responsible and aware, it is very difficult to have the best of what you want. To put it philosophically, "An unexamined life is not worth living."

When you *internalize*, you perform a different sort of disservice to yourself. You suppress and swallow your frustrations, heaping all the blame onto yourself without examining why you failed. You tend to blame your deepest self rather than some action that can be corrected. This results in damaged self-esteem, an inability to act, and can ultimately lead to deep sadness or depression. Victims of domestic violence are often caught in this self-deprecating pattern. It is important for internalizers to understand that *blaming yourself should not be confused with taking responsibility.*

Internalizers often define themselves as losers. They use phrases such as, "I can't do it, so why try? I'm no good at that." "It's all my fault." "I wish I were never born." or the famous line from the movie *Wayne's World,* "I'm not worthy!" When internalizers examine their experiences and failures, their reasoning follows a similarly defeating line of reasoning: "The reason that I'm fat is that I'm weak and have no discipline." If a romantic partner breaks up with an internalizer, he figures, "I'm the sort of person people dump, so I might as well get used to it."

Internalizers can easily get trapped in a vicious circle. A person who feels unwanted may begin to act in an unappealing way, ensuring that no one will want him—a self-fulfilling prophecy.

However, all is not lost. It's possible to interrupt and eventually break these vicious circles by recognizing self-sabotaging thoughts and being willing to examine this thinking in a safe environment, or even in therapy. Once such negative energy begins to be released, held up, and scrutinized, the internalizer begins to take responsibility for making positive internal investigations. Again, understand that by internalizing, you are not taking responsibility—but simply blaming yourself instead of another.

This is not about beating yourself up for the mistakes of your past. Remember that blaming yourself, when inappropriate, can be as destructive as blaming someone or something else. Successful recognition comes from carefully examining your patterns, not placing blame on anyone or anything, but instead looking for the motivations underlying those mistakes in order to correct them in the future.

Compare blame to responsibility and you'll find that *blame looks backward and gets stuck. Responsibility is inherently forward-looking. It asks: Where do we go from here?*

Remember whether you're blaming yourself or others (internalizing or externalizing), you're still using blame to avoid responsibility. The following exercise can help you figure out how to stop blaming and start moving ahead.

EXERCISE 1

Separating Blame From Responsibility

Over the next three weeks, write down at least three situations where you blame yourself or another person (or event) when you should be taking responsibility. Notice how you phrase these situations.

EXAMPLE

Instead of saying, *"My husband left because I was lousy in bed—I've always been lousy in bed . . ."*

Try this: *"I wasn't compatible with my husband, and as a result, our sex life suffered. In my next relationship, I'll pay more attention to the relationship in the very beginning stages and try to look for patterns. And I want to make sure we're sexually compatible."*

Instead of saying: *"I'm destined to be fat. I admit it. Around food, I'm weak and have no discipline. I see food and it seduces me. As far as working out— that's for thin people."*

Try this: *"I'm overweight because I eat many more calories than I burn each day. If I wanted to lose weight, I would be on a program to lower my calorie and fat intake. I should also include some type of fitness program—simply walking would be a good start."*

Write down three of your own examples:

1. Instead of saying what I usually say about (fill in your situation):

   I'll say this:

2. Instead of saying what I usually say about (fill in your situation):

   I'll say this:

3. Instead of saying what I usually say about (fill in your situation):

   I'll say this:

My Genes Made Me Do It—Another Round
in the Blame Game

You cannot pick up a newspaper or magazine these days without reading a story about the scientific findings on the genetic and/or biological bases for human behavior. Advances in the field have shown that there is a gene, or at least a genetic component, for virtually every trait. There appears to be some real foundation for looking into the genetic influence of addiction to alcohol and drugs—which means, of course, that addictive behavior may be programmed into your chromosomes.

Since the '50s, researchers have argued that many aspects of personality and temperament are inborn. Some babies are just born more or less intense, outgoing, whiny, adventurous, timid, somber, persistent, or expressive—you name the trait.

Where does this take you?

You carry inborn traits with you throughout your life, but they can play out in a variety of ways. For example, an overweight person can tame his or her predilection to weight gain by beginning an exercise program and developing new eating habits. How much of this tendency to weight gain, though, is inherited and how much is personal choice? Looking at research involving identical twins seems to prove the point that *personal choice* makes the difference. One such study showed that twins (who have identical biological makeup) could overcome what some would consider a predisposition to adverse genetics.

For example, let's take the case of identical twin brothers who are both overweight. One is able to lose weight and keep it off; the other stays overweight. Another example takes two brothers, identical twins; one is a homeless alcoholic, and the other is a martial arts expert, health nut, and successful photographer. The conclusion:

Neither temperament nor genetics is destiny. It is not what you are born with, but rather what you do with it, that determines where and how your life will go.

There is more to the biology of addiction, appetites, and cravings than mere genetics, of course. Addiction researchers have proposed that cravings result from an upset in the delicate balance between two chemicals in your brain: dopamine, which gives rise to the "I gotta have it" feeling that makes you crave what you crave, and serotonin, which makes you feel the satisfaction that "I got it." The simplest example would be hunger. When you're hungry, the dopamine level rises, focusing your energy, making you more alert, helping you learn, and making you more active. When you eat, the level of serotonin rises, which makes you feel satisfied, less alert, even drowsy. (There are certain foods that counteract this notion, but primarily this is the case.)

In his book, *The Craving Brain,* Dr. Ronald Ruden uses the term "bio-balance" for when your brain achieves a state of harmony between both dopamine and serotonin. Dr. Ruden reasons that destructive addictions might be brought under control by altering brain chemistry, thus allowing for more access to "bio-balance."

Some day soon, scientists hope to form an even more complete picture of how the brain works. They imagine a day when someone who is genetically predisposed to alcoholism can be identified early and will be able to take preventive measures to curb the devastating effects of the condition. Family history still serves as the best indicator of addictive behavior. If you have a close relative or a parent with such a problem, you already know it. In fact, you have probably already suffered some of the consequences.

So, what does the fact that so many of the traits that make you who you are seem to be based in biology and heredity have to do with responsibility? Doesn't a gene pool absolve you of all responsibility?

Of course, there are people who insist that biology explains and excuses all good and bad behavior. I would say that knowing as much as possible about your biology (and family history) leads to an entirely different conclusion: *You can take responsibility for the knowledge and make it work for you.*

Having access to such important information, like whether you're predisposed to alcoholism, is an immensely useful tool in your quest for self-knowledge. It would be foolish to ignore anything that helps you to know yourself more fully and avoid the potential booby traps in your life. This knowledge is not a life sentence—it is a way to make your life better. It gives you a personal barometer so you know what to avoid and what to embrace. It helps you chart a smarter course.

Knowing yourself and being conscious of your personal circumstances and predisposition is the first step in taking responsibility for yourself and what happens to you. Let me stress this point again: Blaming others or blaming genes for your behavior is a step backward and takes away the opportunity for growth and choice. Much valuable energy is lost on blaming.

Holding others responsible for our failures or successes is the road to helplessness. You can't change other people, you can only change yourself and the way you relate and respond to people.

The Higher Authority—Two Views

The majority of the world population believes in some form of God, deity, or a higher authority. Within many of these beliefs exists some level of predeterminism—that one's life is already mapped out, and all one has to do is follow the course and live it out. People of this belief feel they are at the mercy of forces they believe are greater than they are.

However, others who also believe in a deity feel differently: they do not feel they are bound to the "will" of a higher authority or the call of a destiny and instead feel they are free to make choices and to go in any direction.

There are instances when faith can be misused, misapplied, or misplaced. A common way this misuse manifests itself is in language, in which excuses can be disguised as belief:

"If God had wanted it to work out, it would have."
"It's in the stars; there's nothing I can do about it."

When you use language like this, you surrender responsibility to yourself, for yourself.

At other times, "destiny" or the works of a higher authority can intervene and be misunderstood. The following story helps to illustrate this point:

A priest lived in a small town in a valley where a storm was approaching. Flood warnings were announced and the town was evacuated. As the priest's neighbors were leaving their house, they offered him a ride out of town. "I'll be fine," said the priest. "God will take care of me." So the priest stayed in his house. It rained for two days. The streets were flooded and eventually the whole first floor of the priest's house was under by water. He went to the second floor for protection from the flood.

Rescue workers in a rowboat came by and told the priest they would help him out before the waters rose even higher. "I'll be fine," the priest said. "God will take care of me." The workers had no choice but to leave him there.

It kept raining and the waters rose even higher, so much so that the priest had to go up on his roof. A helicopter flying over the disaster area spotted him and a rescue worker dropped a ladder to pick him up. "I'm fine," the priest shouted as he waved them away. "God will take care of me." That night, it rained even more. The waters rose and the priest drowned.

When he arrived in heaven and stood face-to-face with God, the priest demanded: "What happened? I thought you were going to take care of me." God replied: "I kept my promise, I did take care of you! I sent people to save you three times."

I was reading an interview with famous exercise guru Jack LaLanne, which I believe sums it up: "Do you know there are more fat people than there's ever been in our history? It's terrible. People who don't eat right, don't exercise. They drink, then go to church, and then it's 'Dear God, dear God! Please help me with this. Please give me that.' Hey, God is not going to do a thing for you. You do it. He gives you the power to do it. Listen, in the sixty-eight years I've been doing this, I've never heard Jesus knocking on my door at five in the morning saying, 'Jack, I'll work out for you today.'"

Be aware of what has come to help and/or offer you advice—and take it. Responsibility also means improving your life by seizing those golden moments when you are given a gift of knowledge, of life, or of opportunity. Be careful not to allow ideas of predetermination stop you from pursuing your goals.

The Victim—No More "Poor Me"

As discussed previously, I believe there are very few true victims. The victim I'm talking about here usually suffers from the "Poor Me" syndrome. Again, this is not to say you haven't had some unfortunate incident befall you, that put you in an undesirable place. But remember: You may not be responsible for what happened to you, but you are responsible for how you react to that situation. Think of yourself as a victim, and you weaken yourself or become trapped and doomed to staying a victim for the rest of your life. There are times when you feel desperate and helpless, but the truth is that you probably have more choices to rescue yourself than you may at first believe. When faced with difficulties or setbacks, many people think or say, "This always happens to me." You hear variations of it all the time: "I do my job, but I never get the promotions . . ." "My kids are always taking advantage of me . . ." "I have the ideas, but I always get shafted when the deal is put together." Here are other familiar complaints:

▸ "My boss is out to get me."
▸ "The job market is just terrible right now."
▸ "You never listen to me."
▸ "You never talk to me."
▸ "No one appreciates me."
▸ "If there's a rotten job out there, I'll be hired for it."

The "Poor Me" reaction is both positive and negative. On the one hand, voicing the opinion, "This always happens to me" shows an awareness of a negative and repetitive pattern; This is positive. On the other hand, you're saying you exert no control or play no active part in the event. This is a negative. The accompanying beliefs are that you are passive, hamstrung, a victim—someone to whom things "just happen." There's a feeling of helplessness communicated in the phrase.

Negative patterns like "Poor Me" result from the way you run your life, and the habits you get into in your efforts to avoid discomfort. The funny thing is, although you may *think* you're avoiding difficulty and dis-comfort through these habits, you are, in fact, often compounding them.

But, as I've said before, if you can create, you can also destroy. A child knocking down a block tower he has built is aware of this maxim. He can build, he can destroy, and he can then rebuild again. A conscious, aware adult who has done her homework, and decides where she wants to go, can also build a healthier pattern—a better structure to hang her life on.

Inevitably, an egg will break. There's a gap between knowing this and believing yourself capable of recreating yourself. You must believe you have the agency and the power to do all this creating and breaking and recreating again, a facility that psychologist Albert Bandura calls "self-efficacy." Some events in life may sap you of this belief, but hang in there and allow yourself to rediscover it.

This is not to say that there are no victims in life or situations in which people are victimized. But there are very few pure victims, and to define yourself as one is self-defeating from the start. Do you really want to hand the reins of your destiny completely over to someone or something else by putting yourself in the position of asking for pity, not power?

But wait, you may argue. Some people are dealt luckier hands than others in life. Some are smarter, some are taller, some are more gorgeous, some are richer. Some are born on third base without much of a run to home plate. Bad things, tragedies, and illness do sometimes happen to people who are responsible, work hard, and live a fulfilling life. My answer to that is, no one lives a life free of pain and struggle, though you may sometimes be tempted to think that others have it easier. Luck plays a role for all of us, but it plays a smaller role than many people imagine. You can either bemoan that fact or move on and work with what you've got. You have to play the hand you're dealt.

Look at someone like Christopher Reeve, the *Superman* actor who was paralyzed after a terrible equestrian accident. Reeve could have blamed himself for not falling correctly, or crumbled into a ball of self-pity, but instead, he responded in a very impressive and valiant way. He continues to perform and direct films, participate in charitable foundations, and grow spiritually.

Consider a less severe example from my own life: For more than 18 months, I worked night and day to build an Internet company and it was going well. We attracted top industry talent and grew to a staff of more than 40—the site was even voted one of the top in its field.

Unfortunately, the company ran out of money and I had to let our hard-working staff go then regroup and look for new financing. Who should bear the blame? Well, for one thing, the floundering market didn't help.

Second, ours was a content site, and even though the information was excellent, that didn't make it any easier because content companies had fallen out of favor with the market. So, even though everyone worked very hard to create a great product, I still could not secure funding.

It was tempting to think, "Poor me . . . caught in a new industry in a bad market period." Was it "bad luck" or "bad timing?" To some degree, it was both. But some of our competitors, who had not built anything near to the quality and success that our team had built, were able to raise 20 times the amount of money we did. I even started to think that I didn't stand a chance—"I just wasn't lucky enough, those big successes just don't happen to people like me."

Again, if I look carefully at the situation and analyze it, I can see what might have prevented our company from having to start over. I made a choice to move forward with the project even though I had not secured "blue chip" venture financing. I made a choice to pursue the content space online, even though I knew that it was a difficult task. I made a choice to start the company in New York, when I knew that most financing opportunities were in San Francisco. The bottom line is that I'd had choices, and even though I did my best under the circumstances I selected, I was ultimately responsible for the end results.

I reminded myself of something while this was going on: You can improve your responses even when the worst possible events befall you. I knew that "Poor Me" thinking would get me nowhere in rebuilding a successful business. I also learned that to break a negative pattern like "Poor Me," you have to believe you have the ability to do it.

Try this Exercise:

EXERCISE 2

Breaking the "Poor Me" Pattern, Part 1

Altering the language you use every day to tell your story and to express your frustrations can help you change how you take responsibility and behave. Language shapes the way you view things, just as your view of thing shapes the way you talk about them. It goes back and forth, and you have to jump in somewhere. It may be easier, in some ways, to redo your language before you redo your thoughts. It helps when you talk about your life with yourself as the subject, the primary actor, and the cause of many of the events.

When you're ready to take responsibility for your life, nothing is more useful than to begin by speaking about your place in the universe in a different way. The words you use can influence the way you think, and vice versa. Try this:

When discussing failures, setbacks, disappointments, or mistakes, here's a way to change the "Poor Me" trap: Begin your sentences with the word, "I." It's an exercise that will help. Many physiologists and therapists suggest that by just using "I" statements when talking and discussing issues, you can modify your behavior affirmatively. Some examples: "I often put myself in this position." And, "I tend to do (fill in the blank) when the going gets rough." Of course, you don't want to say, "I'm always at the short end of the stick." Turn the sentiment around to see what you may be doing wrong *so that you can correct it.*

Think of something you did today. Describe it by beginning your sentences with the word "I" and following it with an *action verb* to show that "I did" something or "I am doing something," rather than using a form of the verb "to be" such as "I am." By using "to be" you describe yourself in passive terms.

Let's take an example. A commonly heard excuse is, "I'm really busy." You're apt to offer this up as a reason for not completing a project on time for a client, or to a friend you have not called back or seen for a while. You may be, in fact, extremely busy. A lot of people are these days, but is that the real reason? Busy people need to prioritize, so the truth of the situation might be closer to: "I didn't prioritize correctly. I put it off for too long," which is what you might say to a boss or a client. They might even find your honesty and candor refreshing.

To a friend, you could say: "I forgot to call you. I apologize and didn't mean to put you off. But please don't hesitate to call me again if you haven't heard from me. I always love to hear from you." Another approach, both proactive and responsible would be: "I want to have a really good talk with you when I have enough time to focus completely. Let's set a time and a day next week when we can do that. I'll put it on the top of my list for that day."

When you put the word "me" at the end of your sentence rather than an "I" at the beginning, you confirm your passivity and helplessness and allow a negative pattern to continue. Think what a difference it makes when you change, "My boss is screwing me" *to* "I choose to stay in this job despite the fact that my boss undermines my authority." The first keeps you in the victim state. The second opens up a whole line of inquiry and potential action. Why do I choose to stay in this job? What can I do to change that? Or another example: You can change, "My boyfriend is always picking fights with me," to "I allow my boyfriend to push the buttons that get me into arguments. By responding angrily, I encourage him."

Starting sentences with "I" opens the gate to self-reflection, and to recognition of your role in whatever is making you unhappy. It is the first step toward the development of a new positive pattern, that of individual responsibility.

EXERCISE 3
Breaking the "Poor Me" Pattern, Part 2

Write down five situations you've been involved in—a project, relationship, or event that did not go according to plan—whether or not you think it was your fault. After you've written down each event, read through it again. When you get to the part about what went wrong or where the problem occurred, rephrase it so that *you're the one who is ultimately responsible.* Don't place any blame on another person, luck, connections, etc.

Diana's story illustrates what I mean. Her "Poor Me" issues stem from the kind of man she believes she attracts. She said:

"My relationship with Harry, my first husband, was doomed from the beginning. All he really wanted was to be taken care of and it didn't matter who was taking care of him as long as it was done. He was verbally abusive for years, and constantly cheated on me. Harry was, and still is, a world class jerk."

Okay, now let's transform this into an "I" statement:

"I married Harry even though I knew the marriage was doomed from the start. I really wanted to be married, so I overlooked many of his negative characteristics. I made myself believe he'd grow out of them over the years. I allowed Harry to verbally abuse me because I was not ready to leave the relationship—it was just too difficult at the time. I really wanted to make things work. Staying there was my choice, and I understand that now. For the same reasons, I also chose not to confront Harry about his cheating on me. I guess I was just afraid to be alone."

Play the Cards You're Dealt and Make It a Winning Hand!

Recent history is full of examples of people who have overcome huge odds to achieve great success in life. What successful people share, rather than some specific inborn talent or ability, is the ability to turn negatives into positives, liabilities into assets. This ability is cultivated or learned and practiced. Steven J. Hawking, is one of the world's best-known physicists, and a best-selling author, despite his serious physical disabilities. Stevie Wonder, despite his blindness, is arguably one of the best (and one of the richest) songwriters of the century. In spite of their physical challenges, it seems that these two men were more deeply tuned in to their strengths, and pursued them with zeal and passion. They focused on what they could do, not on what they could not, and went forward from there. Beethoven did not let his deafness later in life keep him from composing and sharing the music he heard in his head.

You might be thinking to yourself: "I've heard all of this before. All these great people have overcome these incredible odds—blah, blah, blah. I'm not Steven J. Hawking or Stevie Wonder, and I don't have their great talents. I'm just Suzie Reynolds or Tom Smith. It's just too much." Many times, it seems overwhelming, but to move forward, grow, and break patterns, you must learn how to respond positively under adverse or negative situations, and *move beyond your perceived limitations*. This makes you responsible for yourself.

In other words—deal with it.

James Earl Jones is a great example of someone who dealt brilliantly with adversity—someone who made lemons out of lemonade. Known as one of the most recognizable voices in the world, and sometimes referred to as "The Voice of America," he actually stuttered as a child. He was so deeply ashamed of this speech impediment that he remained virtually mute from the age of 8 to 14. One day, a teacher accused the teenage Jones of plagiarizing a poem and challenged him to read it aloud in front of the class. Jones was so infuriated at the accusation, he rose to the occasion. Suddenly the words flowed freely and smoothly from his mouth.

In the process, the young Jones discovered that reciting the written word was safe from his stutter, so he began devouring the classics. Not only did he overcome his stutter and become a great actor seen in more than 120 films, but also he became renown for his voice, the very thing that plagued him in his youth. That voice has been heard worldwide on the stage, in *Star Wars*, *The Lion King*, and, of course, "This is CNN" and "Welcome to Verizon."

The Avoider—Turning Your Back on Responsibility

Some people just don't like confrontation and will go to great lengths to avoid discussing or even arguing about problems. Sandy, for example, has made such avoidance a way of life. A personal trainer in New York, Sandy is good at what she does and has many regular clients, even some celebrities. She had been dating William for about a year and she cared about him a lot. The problem was that Sandy was basically angry about William's lack of commitment to the relationship but she wouldn't face up to it—to herself or to him. He was constantly reminding her that he wasn't ready to marry and how happy he was with the way things were. When William tried to discuss why he wouldn't marry, Sandy would move onto another subject. She believed that if she didn't hear what William was saying, she wouldn't have to deal with the consequences.

Meanwhile, she started dating one of her clients and didn't tell William. Eventually, William found out and used the excuse of her "infidelity" to break up with Sandy. Then Sandy's client, who was never committed to her in the first place, lost interest and left her too.

With both men gone, Sandy continues to avoid the issue of how she smothers intimacy by not talking about what counts, when it counts. She thinks, "it's simpler" and "less complicated" to turn her back on the reality of who feels what, rather than facing it.

The following are a few Avoider phrases to look for:

▸ "What problem? Everything's just great."

▸ "What's there to talk about?"

▸ "I'm too busy to talk about this right now."

▸ "If I don't ask, I won't know. Then I don't have to worry about it."

Avoiders are guilty of a version of *self-deception.*

Most of us have been guilty of self-deception at some time or another. You may have done something or felt something you don't want to admit to—not to yourself and not to others. At the most extreme, there's the criminal who may deny responsibility for a crime he committed, and he may actually get away with deceiving the authorities. In some cases, he may even believe the lies he tells and deceive himself.

Self-deception, psychologists have noted for years, is a powerful force. Dr. Anthony Greenwald, a psychologist at the University of Washington, suggested that the mind, at times, works like a totalitarian state, not unlike the one depicted in George Orwell's *1984.* The flow of information is kept under very tight control, so that we are able to conceal or censor unpleasant realities, even to ourselves. People often convince themselves that they are responsible for the good outcomes, but not the bad ones. This is why the saying "success has many fathers, but failure is an orphan," rings so true.

Anna Freud, Sigmund's daughter and also a psychoanalyst, called the ways in which we "protect" ourselves from unpleasant realities, "ego defense mechanisms." Two of the most common defense mechanisms are *repression* and *denial.*

Some of these terms have become part of our everyday vocabulary. People throw them around in normal conversation, like, "My boyfriend is in total denial about our relationship."

It goes deeper. With repression, the ego excludes from consciousness whatever it cannot accept. Difficult experiences are shoved into the unconscious mind—swept under the rug. The most common example is that of a childhood trauma, such as sexual abuse, where the person cannot process the pain and, instead, represses it or "forgets."

Denial occurs when you *refuse* to acknowledge the very existence of an event or problem. For example, a marriage may be deeply troubled because of spousal abuse, but the person being abused denies the madness of it—fearing divorce more than physical pain and humiliation within the marriage. A man is consistently fired from his jobs, but then denies his responsibility in this repetitive career event. A woman complains that her husband is cold and uninterested in her sexually, but she denies how she manages to start some sort of fight with him every night before going to bed.

There are other ego defense mechanisms that you may use to get through difficult times. *Rationalization* means you give yourself plausible explanations for how you behaved. In other words, you devise excuses to make yourself feel you're right. *Intellectualization* happens when you avoid painful emotional awareness of problems by analyzing them too abstractly. For example, a smoker might say: "I need one vice, so it's cigarettes." Or, "My grandfather smoked and he lived to be 95," instead of saying, "I smoke because I need the nicotine to feel good," or "Smoking makes me feel in control."

For your purposes, "ego defense mechanisms" are examples of the lengths you go to and the ways you avoid responsibility. Although denial, repression, rationalization, and intellectualization may have their place in protecting you from certain traumas, they're not useful as long-term strategies because they keep you from finding real solutions. The repressed trauma will haunt you in some way. The denied problem will not just go away if you ignore it for long enough. Rationalization and intellectualization keep you from the truth of things, and, therefore, from effective action.

Why do you go to such lengths to avoid seeing the truth and doing something about it? Freud said you do it to protect yourself from anxiety. While this is an understandable goal, I would suggest that you can come up with a much more productive means to relieve yourself of life's inevitable stresses. But I'll get to that later, toward the end of the chapter, when I discuss concrete strategies for taking responsibility, and moving forward to reach your goals.

The following stories illustrate how ego defense mechanisms, like denial and rationalization, affect real life. I call such responsibility-avoiding behaviors "Efforts to Avoid Efforts," or anti-responsible behavior.

The Avoider usually blocks progress through *denial* and *rationalization*. Sometimes you work very hard to avoid the truth of a particular situation, an effort that is completely wasted. In truth, what you may be avoiding is change itself. You prefer the devil you know to the devil you don't. Making that phone call, arranging that meeting, telling your boss or co-worker or loved one how you really feel about a particular situation usually leads to change. You may not feel up to the challenge, but keep in mind, that change requires rethinking, refocusing, and even loss. Paradoxically, *by avoiding uncomfortable situations and not taking responsibility, you're guaranteeing failure, or at the very least, delaying the achievement of your goals.*

Let me begin with Karen to demonstrate what I mean about "anti-responsible" behavior. Karen runs a successful chain of coffee bars on the East Coast. Fred, one of her best friends from college, was her construction manager from the beginning. Fred was a great designer, and his ideas helped shape the business and even make it a success. But he was also consistently late with projects, which was just one of the problems Karen faced with him.

Although Fred was creative with ideas, he wasn't good at seeing a project all the way through, or taking care of the details. As Karen became more successful and sought to expand her business, she began to attract outside investors. She kept Fred on as her designer, even though she was starting to have reservations about his work. She needed someone who was both good at design and good with executing the details, but with what she was paying Fred, she couldn't afford to hire a second person. She frequently nagged Fred to get work done faster, usually to no avail. Fred figured they were friends, and that he was doing Karen a favor working at a substantial discount, and making the coffee bars a success.

Instead of confronting Fred, Karen complained about him bitterly to other people. "Fred screwed up again," Karen would say.

"Then why don't you hire someone else?" a friend would suggest.

"You're right, I should, but I'm too busy with other stuff," Karen would say. "And I don't know any other designers. Fred's a good designer and I owe him."

Karen put herself in a tricky spot, of course, by both denying the situation and by rationalizing Fred's worth. The solution came when outside investors began pressing Karen to get the coffee bars built on time. She finally realized that it was no longer just her money. She had to take herself seriously as a businesswoman. In her mind, she had to fire Fred or lose the business. It was painful, and the friendship was permanently damaged, but Karen felt she had no choice.

Although Karen faced up to the reality that she needed to take action, Fred did not. To this day, he blames Karen for disloyalty, rather than acknowledging that he should have delegated some responsibility for details and schedules to someone else who could do it, and therefore force himself to ask for the right fees to handle large scale projects.

You may recognize yourself in either Karen or Fred. Neither one is a bad person. They are both stuck in a very understandable predicament, one that many of us can relate to. But they both avoided taking steps to find an effective solution—and this is where troubles begin.

The Excuse Maker

Before I learned the strategies in *Breaking the Pattern,* I was at my most creative when it came to making excuses and avoiding moving toward my goals. You, too, can come up with hundreds of clever excuses for not reaching your goals. And many times, the excuses take up more energy than actually getting where you want to go. The trouble is, some excuses are so airtight, that you can talk yourself out of doing anything and avoid accepting responsibility. They sound like:

- ▸ "I'm too tired."
- ▸ "I've got a bad back/shoulder/knee/ankle."
- ▸ "It's too late for me."
- ▸ "I don't have enough time."
- ▸ "I don't know where to begin."
- ▸ "It's just too hard."
- ▸ "Only if I had the right training."
- ▸ "My boss doesn't like me."
- ▸ "I'm too old."
- ▸ "There just wasn't enough time to finish."
- ▸ "I've just been so busy lately."

I offer a word of wisdom about excuse making from a friend who is a recovering alcoholic. He says: "There are a million excuses to pick up a drink again, but no good reason." If you focus on reasons rather than excuses (and really know the difference between the two), you go a long way toward taking responsibility for yourself.

Find an Excuse Buster Instead

You need to come up with persuasive self-talk to counteract your most common justifications for not getting things done. In the goal-planning chapter of this book, which is next, you'll discover the top five excuses that prevent you from moving toward your goal. Meanwhile, in the following Exercise, test the level of your excuse making: Come up with a very specific goal and then create five excuses—make them your best. Then write down your *solutions* to overcome those excuses.

Remember: Always have a back-up "Plan B" when it comes to excuse busting. These alternatives will help motivate you to do what you have to do. For example, if you were planning to go running outside ("Plan A"), but it's raining, your "Plan B" could be to go to an aerobics class, use a track at the gym, or use an exercise videotape in your own home. This type of proactive behavior really helps to accomplish your goals. Without thinking ahead, you leave too many things for chance. And if you really want something bad enough, why coast on excuses and put it off? Make your own choices—don't let them be made for you.

The Counter Puncher

Creating confusion or obfuscating an issue is an effective tactic in avoiding responsible behavior. So when an individual is confronted with a problem, they take an offensive position, that is "counter punching," or hitting offensively with words. By starting a war of words, you immediately take attention away from your own responsibly in a conflict. Counter punchers usually end up walking away *unchanged* (and having learned nothing) from the issues for which they are primarily or partially responsible.

Jenny, a 24-year-old investment banker, had been dating Bill for two years. Jenny was consistently late for their dinner dates, never cleaned up after herself, and worked late almost every night. Whenever Bill would try and explain his feelings, Jenny would start screaming and come up with ten different things that Bill did wrong. Bill would immediately become defensive, get angry, and instead of Jenny taking responsibility, Bill ended up apologizing. As a result, the relationship failed, and Jenny continues to repeat the same pattern with her latest relationship.

Jenny used what she thought to be an asset (her strong verbal skills), as a method of avoiding responsibility to herself, to Bill and to their relationship.

The Ingratiator

"Taking responsibility has to do with telling the truth. I don't mean telling the truth in some sanctimonious, crapola, literal sort of way, but being willing and able to say something stinks when it stinks, and someone doesn't know what he's talking about, and that the emperor has no clothes when he has no clothes," wrote Michael Wolff in his book, *Burn Rate: How I Survived the Gold Rush Years on the Internet.* Wolff touches on another aspect of personal responsibility that can fuel too many engines in big or small business: currying favor, or ingratiation.

Webster's Dictionary defines ingratiate as "to gain favor or favorable acceptance by deliberate effort." Wanting to be appreciated and liked is natural, but it can be done to excess, and to one's own downfall. Ingratiation is an ancient and excellent method of humbling yourself, flattering others—and taking emphasis off the requirements or seriousness of a situation and putting on to the workings of a personality. "You're so good at this, I only wish I could have your ability," an Ingratiator might say to a boss to steer him away from the fact that the work was not done or not done right.

You'll recognize other standard comments from this type when he/she's determined to avoid responsibility:

▸ "Things always seem to go your way. I wish I had it so easy."

▸ "I only did it because I love you."

I think Adam's story illustrates how ingratiation becomes a trap: Adam worked as a partner in a medium-sized New York accounting firm where he enjoyed an excellent relationship with the other partners. They thought Adam was a great guy who always had a ready compliment or a funny joke. The problem was that Adam was a terrible accountant and had been covering it up for years. He missed deadlines, made minor but costly mistakes, and avoided being terminated because he could "make everyone feel good." Finally, Adam blundered in a big way and, as a result, the firm was drawn into a costly legal battle.

Eventually, Adam was terminated, and his percentage of the partnership purchased back by the other partner. He may have relied on his ingratiating style of behavior to get by, but by avoiding responsibility, he failed to care about crucial accounting practices that meant his livelihood; he played at work, rather than applying himself, and he was left jobless.

Often, people use this pattern of behavior because they're unable to communicate their thoughts and feelings, and as a result, lack sincerity. To be truly responsible, you also have to mean what you say. No means no. Yes means yes. It should not be hard to mean what you say, but some people are out of practice. You agree to do things you don't want to do out of a sense of obligation and to avoid conflict. You make dates with acquaintances, relatives, and business associates you don't want to see so as not to hurt their feelings. Sometimes, this backfires and those same people see right through you, dooming the relationship sooner or later. You take jobs or assignments you have no passion for, then drag your feet or do half-baked jobs on them, satisfying no one. You allow people to take advantage of you, allow employees to be late, or allow friends to stand you up. You buy things you don't need so as not to offend the salesman.

Saying "no" can make you feel guilty at first. But when you realize you have the power to say "no," each "yes" becomes much more potent, heartfelt, and conscious. It's the difference between agreeing automatically when your boss asks you to do a task that you don't want to do and saying yes because you want to keep the job. If you like what you're doing for the most part, taking on specific tasks you don't like (for the good of the overall job) is actually *being responsible to your commitment to keep the job* and advance in it. Every job has its "grunt work," and irritations.

The difference may seem subtle, but the second "yes" is more of a choice. Its being conscious and aware of its implications—reaching your goals. And remember, if it doesn't negatively impact your position, you could also say "no."

The Martyr

Another meaningful look into responsibility hinges on your idea of helping others. A martyr typically will suffer for others—sacrifice for the good of another. Lawyer, sailor, and author of *Godforsaken Sea*, Derek Lundy, touched on these components:

"Each person is responsible for every word and act he or she says or does. Almost every human being is a potential torturer and murderer. Our prime responsibility is certainly to avoid those extremes, but also, as much as possible, not to hurt other people at all. We should all take the Hippocratic Oath to do no harm. If we have any energy left over, we can try to do some good as well."

Clearly, Lundy believes in a deep moral component of responsibility. I have to agree. Once you take responsibility for yourself, you're better able to take responsibility for other people. Some people have this turned around. Some people take better care of others than they do of themselves, for whatever reason, perhaps low self-esteem. The typical example is the self-sacrificing mother, who tends to all of her children's needs while ignoring her own. Such an imbalance can lead to problems. There is a reason, for example, why the "emergency procedures" on an airplane advise people flying with small children to first put on their own oxygen mask when there is a loss of cabin pressure; someone who is not breathing cannot properly protect a small child.

People in the so-called "caring" professions such as doctors, nurses, and counselors are to be commended. Many discover that they need to put limits on how much they do for others and not shoulder too much of the burden. Even a very sick person ultimately retains some responsibility, however sad his condition. To deprive a person of that is to rob him of all his power and dignity.

Acceptance is another way of coping with Martyr behavior. Acceptance means swallowing your pride, owning up to your role in events, and taking responsibility for making them better. John is a good case in point to illustrate the connection between acceptance and responsibility.

Every week, John's mother hosts a family get-together at her house in the suburbs. Every week, John dreaded the dinner, but felt obligated to go, and reluctantly made the trip. First, he would bitch and moan all week about how he had to waste his Friday night traveling all the way to his mom's house. The whole train ride, he would fret about the time he was wasting. When he got there, he would constantly look at his watch. Since he resented being there, he would frequently get into arguments with various members of his family. He also resented the fact that he would feel too guilty to enjoy himself if he did not show up.

Finally, John experienced one of those "Aha!" moments when people see things clearly at long last. He realized that it was his own decision to go to his mother's house for dinner. No one was holding a gun to his head. John accepted the fact that he went there of his own free will. He also realized that his own resentment fueled much of the conflict and tension he so disliked.

The next week, John called his mother and said: "I'm not coming to dinner this week. I'm too busy and I'm not in a good state of mind." His mother was disappointed, but the world did not come to an end. His family did not disown him. After not going for a few weeks, John realized that he missed it a little. He missed his mother's cooking and missed being with his family. He even missed the train ride, which he realized gave him an opportunity to reflect on his work. He decided he would go every other week, but the experience would never be associated with the same dread again. He had *accepted his own responsibility* for making the experience unpleasant. When the experience became a choice rather than an obligation, it took on a whole new light in his eyes. The dinners became rewarding and fun.

Awareness and acceptance are essential for creating significant change in your life. It may be that you decide you do not want to change. Let's say you go into business with a friend who is fun to be around, but not as hardworking or as results-oriented as another partner might be. But you enjoy working with this person. If your desire for a fun working environment outweighs your desire to be extremely successful, that's fine, as long as you identify your priorities and accept the consequences of your choices.

A friend of mine is a classical violinist who has played with some of the best orchestras in the country. He devoted much of his young life to playing the violin, and became so successful at it that he was frequently on the road, touring to various cities, and making a good deal of money. At a certain point, he was offered a spot in one of the most prestigious orchestras in the country, which would have required even more traveling. He had recently married, and his wife was expecting their first child.

At this crossroads, he made the decision that spending time with his family was more important to him. He took a job as a leader of a smaller, less prestigious orchestra, one that allowed him to stay closer to home. Some of his colleagues thought he was crazy for sacrificing his career in the way he they thought he had. But as he told me, he had never been happier. He felt he had managed to get the best of both worlds.

Responsibility and Taking Control, No Matter What Your Type

I want to make clear to you that taking responsibility is not about anything except taking control and getting results. Far from hemming you in, taking responsibility is profoundly liberating. But how do you go about taking responsibility?

One way is by doing it little by little. The funny thing about taking responsibility/control is that once you do it in some small way in one area of your life, it can gradually become a pattern that will impact the other areas of your life. *It is self-empowerment running the great race, not running on empty.* A study on women and investing affirms this idea by revealing that women who do not see themselves as being in control of their lives are less likely to exercise any control over their financial interests. Women who see themselves as victims of circumstances are less likely to make regular contributions to savings accounts, regardless of age, income level, or marital status. My conclusion: Don't let this happen to you. Instead, believe you have control over your life, be responsible for it, and take the first small step toward change!

Responsibility and Your Surroundings

To a large extent and within your means, you control the environment you function in. You can choose to be with people who bring out the best in you. Or not. If you're trying to stop drinking, but continue to surround yourself with friends who make alcohol a requisite for a good time, I'd have to question your commitment to quitting. If you're trying to lose weight, don't get a job in a bakery. No matter what the problem behavior or addiction (smoking, drinking, overeating, or drugs), *environment* can contribute to both the problem and the solution.

Here are some do's and don'ts:

▶ Remove from your home any reminders or temptations of the behavior you want to change.

▶ Leave places where other people are engaging in that behavior.

▶ Put things around your home and workplace that remind you to avoid that behavior.

▶ Avoid people with whom you once engaged in the behavior.

Taking responsibility for breaking patterns can begin with a change in your environment.

Instead of: *"I need to lose 20 pounds. I'm determined to stop snacking and overeating."*

Try this: *"I will not buy candy and bring it into the house, telling myself it's for the kids."*

Or this: *"Pasta is one of my biggest weaknesses. The next time someone suggests eating at an Italian restaurant, I'll recommend another place or make sure there are low-fat, low-calorie meals on the menu to choose from."*

Being responsible for yourself indicates not only who you are but where you are.

Taking Responsibility and Modifying Behavior

Pick a behavior, perhaps out of one or more of the types I've outlined previously, that you want to modify or change. Write down five things that facilitate or help trigger the behavior, and the changes you will make to avoid putting yourself in compromising situations.

Behavior:

Triggers:

    1.

    2.

    3.

    4.

    5.

Changes:

    1.

    2.

    3.

    4.

    5.

Reaching "Aha!"

Everything you've done up to now (or has happened to you) is an "experience." Applying the concepts of taking responsibility is a powerful way to prevent you from looking at those experiences through tinted glasses and seeing either an idealized or a tragic view.

I've offered you a good hard look at what responsibility means, so now you're ready to go back to the personal histories you wrote out in Chapter 2 (page 38). Try to see your patterns as they truly are. It takes years to develop them, and many are deeply ingrained. But it takes only a moment to decide to make a change, or what I like to call experiencing an "Aha!" moment.

This is not the same as the trigger moment. (A trigger is an event that forces you to realize you want to make a significant change in your life.) *The Aha! moment lets you see how that change will be made.* You catch sight of the light at the end of the tunnel, and with it, the path toward reaching your dreams becomes clear.

For example, if you're dumped in a romantic relationship, you're likely to engage in a significant amount of self-reflection. You may decide you never want to feel this bad again and that something has to change. That's a catalyst or a trigger. The Aha! moment comes when you realize how to change your negative patterns. There's potential to see your responsibility in how the relationship failed. You might also gain insight into how to start the next one with a better sense of yourself. And, just as importantly, you'll develop a plan. Sometimes these Aha! moments strike you out of the blue, but there are ways you can help the process along. By learning and putting into practice the next Principle, you will get the ball rolling.

Summing Up

- You're the only one responsible for your actions—you make the choices that control your life. Responsibility comes from confronting and dealing with the issues (minor and major) that come your way.

- Blaming others or blaming genes for your behavior is a step backward and takes away opportunity for growth and choice. Blaming wastes enormous amounts of valuable energy.

- Being responsible for your own life means you are not bound to predetermined ideas of what your life should be. You're free enough to make choices and go in any direction.

- You may not be responsible for what happens to you, but you are responsible for how you react to what happens to you. Think of yourself as a victim, and you weaken yourself.

- To move forward, grow, and break patterns, you must learn how to respond positively under adverse or negative situations and move beyond your perceived limitations. This makes you responsible for yourself.

- Focus on the reasons you are not breaking your patterns/meeting your goals/finding satisfaction in how you've made your life, rather than on the excuses you make for staying stuck. When you know the difference between the two and apply it, you go a long way toward taking responsibility for yourself.

- To be truly responsible, you have to mean what you say and say what you mean.

PATTERNS

FAILURE

RESPONSIBILITY

GOALS

ACHIEVEMENT

CHAPTER FIVE

What Makes
A Goal A Goal?

In the long run, men hit only what they aim at.
—Henry Thoreau

*If you set high goals for yourself, and every day continue to reflect
on them, step by step, you will be more focused
and make yourself a better human being.*
—Konosuke Matsushita, CEO of Matsushita Electric

Society seems to have been designed to dull your dreams and sensibilities. In childhood, you could dream abundantly and fancifully about what might or might not happen. Your imagination seemed limitless—you were even encouraged to fantasize, create, and spin dreams. But as an adult, your efforts to make dreams come true are often met with resistance, doubt, or criticism. Or, others attempt to impose limitations on you. You may have internalized those doubts and negativity and, out of fear of humiliation and failure, learned to keep your dreams under wraps, concealed sometimes even to yourself. Or, you stop yourself from taking the leap. To break the pattern and unleash your true potential, recapture some of that lost ability to dream! Unearth the visionary inside you.

The fifth century philosopher Confucius declared that wisdom is "when you know a thing, to recognize that you know it, and when you do not know a thing, to recognize that you do not know it." So, while creating your dream, maintain the ability to see yourself and the state of your circumstances practically and clearly. Dreams can be wonderful and energizing, but it takes *discipline* to make them real. Let's meet that head-on.

As an adult, you need to dream realistically and wisely. This wisdom is a combination of tapping into your youthful ingenuity and your innate ability to come up with innovative solutions, tempered by your ability to modify those ideas with the experiences, insights, and principles you've picked up along the way. In adulthood, dreaming is a good start, but it is only the beginning. That beginning leads us to *goals or passions* and more importantly, to goal planning.

What is Goal Planning?

> *I always achieve my goals because I don't quit,*
> *and I have a plan.*
> —Sam LeFrak, billionaire real-estate developer

"When I was growing up, a guy across the street had a Volkswagen Bug. He really wanted to make it into a Porsche. He spent all of his spare money and time accessorizing this VW, making it look and sound loud. By the time he was done, he did not have a Porsche. He had a loud, ugly VW. You've got to be careful choosing what you're going to do. Once you pick something you really care about, and it's a worthwhile thing to do, then you can kind of forget about it and just work at it. *The dedication just comes naturally*," says Steve Jobs, CEO of Apple Computers. Still, many people choose the path of least resistance. Rather than pursue a goal, they take whatever is at hand or whatever comes up, then try to fit themselves into whatever opportunity presents itself.

You can do this in terms of career. You can also do it in your relationships and with your health. It's not the job you want, but you take it because it's better than nothing. You're not really happy with the person you've committed to, but he or she has always been there.

Goal planning can be tricky business. You don't want to err too far on the side of being unrealistic, like the fool Steve Jobs described who wanted to remake his VW into a Porsche. On the other hand, you don't want to err by setting your sights too low, spending a lifetime underachieving, only to end up wondering "what if . . ." you really had applied yourself.

I'm going to propose that life is not such a game of wait-and-see. Your goals, thankfully, are in your hands and are not a matter of chance. I propose that rather than "making do" with whatever presents itself, you instead dare to take a proactive role in creating the world that lives in your dreams. It will not be handed to you. It will not coincidentally materialize if you think about it long enough and hard enough. *It begins with knowing what you want.* Then you have to really want it enough to plan for it, and yes, work for it, sometimes over a long period of time. You also have to be careful, literally, *full of care* about what you want. You have to ponder it, then be clear that you want it badly enough to put a committed effort into making it happen—to sacrifice other more fleeting pleasures. And you will make sacrifices because anything worth having usually involves some struggle. Then, after all of this dreaming, soul-searching, deciding, and steeling of your resolve, you must remember that this is only the beginning—you need a plan.

Why You Need Goal Planning

The focus of the fourth Principle is *Goal Planning* rather than the more familiar phrase "goal setting." Goal setting is something almost everyone engages in to some extent. You can *imagine* a goal and how to make it happen. Or, if you're really ambitious, you can *write* an annual list of goals at New Year's or on your birthday, stick the list in a drawer, and forget about what's on it. For people who choose this method, goal setting is a one-time proposition.

But don't misunderstand me—writing down your goals and putting the list in a drawer is still better than not having any goals at all. You set the goal, but didn't necessarily plot the course to reach it. The thing is, sometimes, what you think of as goal setting amounts to little more than a wish list.

Goal planning, on the other hand, is a much more comprehensive, more intensive, and less fleeting affair. You not only write down a goal, but also outline the steps you'll take to reach it. You devise a thorough plan of attack, complete with contingencies of every sort, and then track your progress, consistently and thoughtfully. Goal planning includes self-monitoring and follow through.

As you'll see below, there's hard evidence that active goal setting and planning for both the short- and long-term lead to higher achievement. High achievement is not something that happens to anyone by accident. It is planned for, visualized, and pursued relentlessly. If you don't set a goal that tells you where you want to go, you could easily end up someplace else. By understanding this Principle, you will embark on the path of defining, visualizing, planning for, and eventually attaining goals and breaking your patterns.

Goals and Risk

I'm not going to sugarcoat the message: It's both brave and risky to have a goal. To have a goal is to admit to wanting something; and to yearn for something implies vulnerability, which is not necessarily a bad thing. It opens you up to the possibility of disappointment, failure, and rejection, which you might be inclined to fear. But having a goal is also a tremendous step in being responsible to yourself. When you actually tell people about your goals, you make the goals that much more real by giving yourself something to live up to, but you also become that much more vulnerable.

Suzanne Yalof, author of *Getting Over John Doe*, said "The biggest chance I ever took was when I said to my fiancé on our fourth date, 'I want to get married and have children eventually and if you don't, then let's move on.' I can't believe he went out with me again—he still teases me."

While she certainly risked rejection by her future husband when she laid her cards on the table so early in their relationship, she also took responsibility for her relationship and its direction.

But, the alternative is worse. To be mired in less-than-ideal circumstances for your one and only life (as far as we know), is to suffer a loss of dreams, which is a crippling condition.

Let me assure you: A goal doesn't have to be something extraordinary or marvelous. It can simply be wanting to make a family, or getting a new car every two years, or getting a promotion at work. Also, don't be intimidated into thinking you must have a goal that is perceived by others as dynamic or extraordinary. You might decide to retire from a busy life and relax more, do a little volunteer work, go back to school, or spend more time with relatives—or even become a couch potato for a little while. You might not want to make any decision right now. That's also OK. Just be clear that this is what you want.

Reaching your goals is not about gambling, that is, unless your goal is to win $1 million in the slot machines in Las Vegas. Getting to your goals is not a matter of random chance no matter how hard you blow on the dice and pray. Getting to your goals requires techniques that greatly improve your chances of achieving. This chapter takes you through the steps, starting with first stages of goal planning.

What Makes a Good Goal?

An easy way to remember how to ensure your goal will be effective is to make it **S.M.A.R.T**:

- ▸ **S**pecific and clearly defined
- ▸ **M**otivating and stimulating
- ▸ **A**chievable (especially in terms of time frame) and honest
- ▸ **R**ewarding
- ▸ **T**actical (have tactics, strategy, and discipline)

Let's take these one by one:

An Effective Goal Is Specific and Clearly Defined

Goals should be specific, so there can be no doubt about your intentions. If you set a goal to "*make more money so I can retire early*," or "*be warmer to my family*," you have not given yourself a clear enough target at which to aim. Your efforts will lack focus and an effective means of measuring their success. A better defined and clearer goal is: "*I'm going to make X amount of money so that I can retire at 45.*"

Most studies show that clear and specific goals with a well-defined target (such as, to retire at 45 years old) are more effective than general "do your best" or "do better" goals. Other studies show that people perform better on tests in which they are asked to find specific objects in a cluttered picture, that is, meeting the goal of finding something specific by filtering out irrelevant information. Specific goals also enable people to use and deal with negative and positive feedback intelligently. When your goal is clear and specific, you can answer questions about your objectives or deal with criticism about your goal from yourself and others.

Let's take the example above on retirement and continue to analyze it:

Having the relatively unclear goal of "making more money to retire early" doesn't *put you on track* or tell you *how far down that track* you are right now. "More" money must be defined with other specifics, such as *when, how much, and through what means?* Having "more" money is difficult to achieve without creating a definite plan. By clearly defining both the long-term goal (to retire by 45) and the interim target (saving/investing/earning "X" dollars per year) and by what means you will earn this money, you're able to evaluate your progress and know whether you are falling short along the way.

Goals vs. Tasks

Goals should not be confused with tasks. Tasks are those little things you do to reach your sub-goals. A task is a piece of work to be accomplished and checked off the list. For example, if you wanted a better job, a related *task* would be to send out resumes to prospective employers. The *goal* is getting a better job.

Performing small tasks has its satisfactions. It gives you the feeling that you're busy and accomplishing things. If you're busy enough, you can avoid doing the more difficult work of thinking out how to approach your goals, which involves a great deal of strategic planning and action. Strangely enough, sometimes people focus on creating and completing tasks to such an extent that it becomes a way of diverting attention and responsibility away from taking action. So, being busy can also be a negative pattern stemming from a lack of confidence and fear of failure.

Understanding Short-Term and Long-Term Goals

Everyone needs both short- and long-term goals. Some short-term goals are based on a sense of urgency (get any job to pay the rent); some are based on recreating, reinventing, or improving your current situation (find an affordable and nice apartment); and lastly, short-term goals are a subset, or *sub-goals* of long-term goals (rent an apartment, and save money so you can eventually purchase a home). All three types are part of life, and shape your life differently.

A Harvard University study showed that people who pursue a set of short-term goals gain encouragement by approaching or attaining their goals more frequently. Short-term goals give you a feeling of control, self-efficacy, and confidence to go on to meet other goals. Long-term goals are essential for "transcendence," the ability to see beyond the immediate situation and its pressures, but their progress can be more difficult to gauge.

Short-term goal planning can do two things—get you a separate goal that's within reach, or, more productively, you may use short term goals as stepping stones to reach the larger goal by breaking it down into manageable pieces or sub-goals. When you reach those smaller goals, you feel your competence and self-efficacy grow. Then you're further encouraged to keep yourself on track.

On the other hand, long-term goals give you motivation, which you need over the long haul to achieve anything substantial. Researchers have found that having distant goals improved and increased people's overall motivation, and *short-term* goals led to more positive expectations of success. The idea is to keep that goal to "lose 30 pounds" or "get a better paying job" as the driving force toward achievement. Another study on goal setting and task performance showed that having long-term goals was associated with better school performance. Students who had goals in the distant future, and who also viewed their efforts in school as part of the process of reaching those goals, maintained higher grade point averages than other students. Long-term goals also help you transcend your immediate situation and any of its unpleasant demands or distracting temptations so you can plan positively for the future—they keep you on track.

Film producer Christine Vachon (*Boys Don't Cry*) illustrated how long-term goals can keep you going in the face of short-term setbacks.

When she first got into film production, she encountered a "really bad period." At that time in New York, there wasn't much work and it was difficult to make a living. She would finish a job in December and not work again until March because of the weather. In Vachon's own words:

> I had just been racking up some nice film production credits, but then suddenly I had the winter ahead of me. So, I scrambled around and got a job as a legal proofreader. I had been doing freelance proofreading for some time. I got on the lobster shift, but I had to go in and train during regular hours and their rules were that you had to dress appropriately. I agonized over it a little bit, and then wore a skirt and a shirt.
>
> When I got there, the woman who ran the proofreading department, who was sort of a little Napoleon, said: "Where do you live?" I told her, Brooklyn. And she said: "How long would it take you to go home and come back?" I said, an hour. She said: "Well, go home and change your blouse because what you are wearing is not appropriate."
>
> So, I walked out and sat down on the steps outside. Every part of me just wanted to leave and not come back, but I wanted the job because I really needed the money so that I could go back to working in film in the spring. I had been a reasonably privileged person, not that I could live off my parents or anything, but I had a strong sense of entitlement. This was my first experience in the real world of work and how you have to swallow a certain amount of pride. So, I had to decide whether to give it up and be furious, or just realize that the job was a means to an end. Big deal, so I have to change my clothes. It was

my first taste of the rule I live by now which is that pragmatism is really the most important thing.

Vachon had many choices here, but she made a choice to stick it out, because of her desire to stay in the film business.

An Effective Goal Is Motivating

Although not every goal is going to be the most exciting or invigorating, you should try tailoring your goals so that you get excited about them. They should be bold, original to you, and should inspire your courage. They should enlarge your life and expand your possibilities. They should increase your happiness and whet your appetite. They should be so daring that they shock people into saying, "You're going to do *what?*" A goal should get your juices flowing and your neurons firing. A goal has to have a certain amount of sexiness, even if a large part of what will get you there is plain, old-fashioned hard work. The objective is to keep your interest and motivation in achieving the goal. If it's boring and uninteresting, it will be much more difficult to obtain.

Remember: *You're the one who has to create and shape your goals so they're interesting and exciting—it may not always come naturally. To stay stimulated, you need to fight two of the weaknesses that routine and commitment can bring up: Procrastination and boredom.*

Procrastination and Boredom

Your time on earth is limited, and in the face of this all-encompassing deadline, you need to put yourself on schedules and set smaller deadlines. A reasonable deadline, whether it is self-imposed or imposed on you by a boss or a teacher, gives you ample time to finish whatever work needs to get done if you use the time wisely. Like a good boss or manager, you need to set reasonable deadlines for yourself so that you can succeed.

But the human animal, some more than others, will procrastinate. You know the story: You squander much of the time allotted for a given task until you're up against a wall and are forced to make an all-out, very pressured effort to complete it, often with bad results. Procrastination is a prime example of a negative pattern, and is also a way of dodging responsibility.

Many of you start to notice your procrastination as students. When you're young and in school, you do not believe that you're responsible for yourself. Most of you have had the experience of waiting until the last minute to study for a test or write a paper, then staying up all night cramming or writing. There is a pleasurable aspect to this self-imposed torture, a certain rush that comes from meeting the emergency and somehow pulling it off. But if you continue this pattern, as you get older, you may find your thrill level decreases, your stress level increases, and that you're left with the rather embarrassing feeling of not having done a very good job.

Is there a way to change procrastination to efficient productivity? Rick is a college student with a paper due at the end of the semester. Since the paper is extensive, he knows he should pick a topic early in the year and start working on the paper about a third of the way through the semester. But when he sits down in front of his computer to start working, he feels bad and has difficulty writing the first paragraph. When he picks the topic, it seems important and he thinks he has a lot to say about it. But now, faced with the blank computer screen, he's unable to translate his thoughts into words.

He thinks about his goals for the paper and realizes they are lofty—to write an outstanding paper with profound insights and extreme lucidity and impress his instructor, thereby demonstrating his superior intellect. The first sentences Rick writes, however, are clunky and trite. Rick becomes depressed and anxious with every subsequent line he puts down. It's not long before he avoids the work.

Now Rick has two problems: the paper itself and his negative feelings about it. To avoid the negative feelings, he avoids the paper. In other words, he procrastinates in order to avoid the reality that the paper might not be all that he dreamed it would be. Instead, he tries to make himself feel better by playing video games with his friends, organizing his CD collection, and going out on the town. He pursues these activities with a certain frantic conviction to keep his anxiety about the deadline suppressed, but of course, the anxiety remains. How could Rick have avoided this problem, or what can he do now to improve the situation? Here's how he went wrong:

- ▸ He put too much emphasis on suppressing his negative feelings.
  Most people in creative pursuits or large writing projects have moments of despair, when they wonder if the work is any good at all. They make themselves feel even worse by anticipating a negative response from teachers, bosses, or critics. Rick avoided the bad feelings by avoiding the project, but that was not the solution. Rick believed, unrealistically, that his idea was great and that he could write about it with ease.

- ▸ He failed to set short-term goals.
  Rick had only the vague, larger goal of writing a brilliant paper. Once he was convinced he was falling short of that, he gave up. He needed to break the bigger project into smaller goals: an outline by a certain date, one written section one week, another the next and so on. He had no concept of the steps he needed to take.

- ▸ He set an unrealistic goal.
  Rick intimidated himself by setting higher standards than he could meet. He could only fail to measure up. Brilliance sometimes happens by accident. It occurs when you focus on making one thing as good as you can—on giving it everything. But deciding to be brilliant from the get-go is putting the cart before the horse. The

same thing is true when you set a goal to find a perfect job or perfect relationship. Perfection is not a realistic goal.

Motivation

Motivation is a mysterious entity. Some people seem to have more of it from the start than others, as if born with it. As you are probably aware, there is an entire industry that has sprung up around teaching motivational skills. But while motivation is certainly a personality trait or characteristic, the most useful thing to know about it is that it comes a lot more easily when it is attached to something meaningful.

In an interview with the father of one of the world's richest men, William Gates Sr. was asked, "If your son had thought he would inherit a fortune from you, would he be as motivated?" Gates Sr. said that "I think it probably is true that growing up in a family of immense wealth, the possibility of a young man being as creative in a business way is sharply reduced . . . my estimate is that if Bill Gates Jr. had grown up in a life of real comfort, the motivation to do what he has done would not have been there."

The most helpful approach for staying motivated is to have clearly defined, challenging, and exciting (but not impossible) goals, for both the short- and long-term, so you know that your efforts are taking you somewhere.

But this is just part of the picture when it comes to motivation. You'll greatly improve your chances of success when you enjoy the process of working toward achievement, not just the end result. That is, when the process is intrinsically rewarding, motivation is likely to follow. When a curious infant picks up objects and examines them, tastes them, and throws them around, he or she is learning, not because of any outside reward, but for the pleasure of learning itself. Later on, children who enjoy learning for learning's sake, not just for reaping good grades or pleasing their parents, are happier and better students.

Let's say your goal is to get married and start a family. You'll probably have better luck if you accept the process of dating as enjoyable and rewarding, rather than if you view it as painful or grueling work. A writer who finds the process of writing rewarding is more likely to keep on writing when the going gets tough (as it inevitably will in any creative pursuit). Weight loss and fitness are difficult examples, since a certain amount of pain, or at least, the limitation or denial of pleasure, is involved in exercise and eating right. Still, many people attain unexpected highs in the pursuit of a fitness goal as they begin to feel stronger and more energetic almost immediately. They feel a sense of pride in their accomplishments along the way.

Many psychologists and social critics have said that we rely too heavily on extrinsic rewards to motivate people. Extrinsic rewards include things like grades in school, paychecks for work, rewards and punishments from parents, and the approval of others. The problem seems to be that people who work purely for external rewards do so with less enthusiasm and efficiency. They come to enjoy the rewards and not the work itself, and are easily tempted to take shortcuts to reach their goal.

To achieve *your* long-term personal goals, you should be driven primarily by intrinsic rewards—that inner fire will provide you with all the motivation you need. But, there's a place for extrinsic rewards as well, especially if you're giving something up, as in the case of addiction. For example, if you want to stop smoking, try treating yourself to a CD or a book with some of the money you would have spent on a $4–$5 pack of cigarettes. This gift to yourself helps reinforce at least one of the benefits of giving up a negative pattern, albeit, not the most important benefit. Setting up a reward system for yourself for not smoking definitely helps in the beginning.

Ultimately, though, the real motivation for quitting smoking should come from within—you can't keep up your motivation by buying CDs forever; the two are only distantly related. A more lasting source of motivation comes from your improved self-esteem, the desire for better health, cleaner lungs, a longer, less illness-plagued life, the chance to view more sunsets, more great art, experiencing more hugs with those you love, having more energy, and the satisfaction from having attained a desired and difficult goal. While perhaps less concrete and tangible, all these are more rewarding in the long run than a room full of CDs.

If your goal is to lose weight, try to visualize the personal rewards that will come with it. Chances are you will feel better and more energetic and have an improved self-image. Feeling more confident and svelte, you will likely be more attractive to people, and date more if you are single, or just have a more fulfilling social and sex life if you are not. Think of those rewards when you are tempted to overeat.

Finally, the best reward for meeting any goal is the sense of achievement, the pride in the accomplishment, and the expanded sense of your own potential that comes when you meet a difficult challenge. When you set, plan for, and meet a goal, you feel more in control and responsible for your life. There is no better feeling.

Envy—Good and Bad for Motivation

It was St. Thomas Aquinas who included envy in his list of the seven deadly sins. Throughout the history of the world, the negative consequences of envy have been illustrated again and again. I could start with the story of Cain and Abel or Milton's depiction of Satan's fall from paradise in *Paradise Lost*, or even Iago's treachery in Shakespeare's *Othello* in which envy is described as the "green-eyed monster." Envy has been the cause of many a man's ruin. No matter how potentially ruinous, envy seems to be a near universal emotion. In Denmark, there is a proverb: "If envy were a fever, all the world would be ill." A common phrase in Bulgaria is: "Other people's eggs have two yolks." Envy may indeed be the root of much of man's unhappiness, and yet it also seems to drive much of human action.

No question about it: There's a dark side to envy. According to the *Oxford English Dictionary*, "envy" comes from the Latin word *invidere*, which means, "to look maliciously upon." *Webster's Dictionary* talks of envy as the painful awareness of an advantage enjoyed by another, and the desire to have the same advantage.

Envy is evident in many aspects of human life. You may envy your neighbor's bigger house or expensive car. You may envy a friend's figure, athletic prowess, or luck—always hoping they lose and you gain or vice versa. The power games that occur in many large corporations are often rooted in feelings of envy for one's superiors or fellow employees. The darker side of envy arises when we not only want what someone else has, but also when we may want to hurt or deprive him or her in the process. Also envy can turn you against yourself. Some people are so overwhelmed by unbearable feelings of envy they become hopeless and withdraw from competition altogether.

Since envy is so much a part of human nature, I've often wondered if it's possible to harness the energy and motivation that comes from it and use it as a positive force? Envy can be a strong and positive motivational tool, even a wake-up call. The Spanish philosopher Gracian once said that nothing "arouses ambition so much as the trumpet blare of another's fame." Vindictive or self-defeating behavior where the idea is to beat others out, goes nowhere, and is all about anger, not achievement. However, *using envy in a relatively benign and harmless way—specifically, by awakening a healthy competitive instinct*—can help you cope with these feelings.

Many titans of the business world have been spurred on by competition, which is the prime motivating force in capitalism. In his autobiography, Lee Iacocca—who became famously successful for rebuilding Chrysler—recounts a longstanding and complicated relationship with his friend and competitor Henry Ford II. That relationship helped drive his success. Bill Gates and Steve Jobs are other rivals in the same industry, both of whom like to win and triumph over the other.

If you take responsibility for yourself, set and carefully plan goals, and are successful in your pursuits, you lose your reason to envy others. In general, pursuing excellence is a way of dealing with envy. Success, or, as the old adage says, "living well," is truly the best revenge.

EXERCISE 1
Taming Your Envy

You must be aware of your envy and its target before you can tame it and make it useful. Therefore, take some time to reflect and focus on the people you envy. Let that envy fuel your motivation.

1. Think about what they have that you covet, and why. Try to be as specific as possible.

2. Are these things truly important to you?

3. If you want those same things for yourself, how would you get them—figure it out?

An Effective Goal Is Achievable and Honest

While your goals should get you excited, they also need to be balanced with a realistic time frame, *self-knowledge* and *planning* what is really *doable*. "I'm going to be elected president next year," or "I'm going to own a recording company in six months," may excite you plenty, but you need to be aware that things don't always happen that way, or that fast.

One of the most common self-defeating behaviors is setting unrealistic goals. A common mistake is to try and "prove everyone else wrong" by over-reaching, then falling on your backside. Set goals that you know in your heart you can, and truly, want to achieve. You have to know and be honest *about your own capabilities*, understand the *nuts and bolts* of the goals you set (whether business or personal) and fit all the details into a *time frame* that's manageable.

Most worthwhile acts take a long time to build and prepare for. A time frame is important. No amount of striving and preparing will get you elected president unless you've made yourself a known candidate with supporters and a platform, way before any campaigning starts during an election year. It takes years, not weeks, to build a business, and even more time to make it profitable. Having a wonderful relationship with a significant other takes time, communication, planning, and hard work—it's not like a romance movie. And if your goal is to lose a great amount of weight and finally keep it off, you must know that weight won't disappear in a few days, or a few weeks.

Be realistic and reduce the futility quotient—make sure you know what you're getting into. You can test for how realistic a goal is by asking yourself the question: "Is it under my control?" Goals like: "I'll get in such great shape, I'll be asked to model on the cover of *Vogue*" or "I'm going to be the president of IBM by the time I'm 40," are lofty, but they require other people to recognize you and take certain actions—actions that are not under your control. You might be in "good enough shape" to be on the cover of *Vogue* or have the skills and experience to be the president of IBM, but it may not be in your control. The approval and admiration of other people is often a byproduct of successfully reaching your goals, but it shouldn't be the primary objective.

It's important to know what skills you actually have. Skills are critical because they help to break patterns and facilitate achievement. A skill is defined as the ability to use your knowledge effectively and readily in performance, or a learned power, which helps you do something competently. Consider your most important skills as the ones you have used effectively in the past. A skill can be a knack for learning languages, fixing anything with a motor, building furniture, being good with computers, listening to people, or assisting others. You can identify your skills by listing and analyzing five of your most important achievements. These achievements should combine personal, spiritual, work, hobbies, etc. Be as specific as possible when preparing this list—don't just state a result, try to come up with the actual accomplishment. From this list of achievements, note if anyone else was involved (to see if there's someone specific who you work well). For each achievement, list which factors motivated or excited you to excel in this situation, and list your exact role. Look at the skill(s) that you used for each one of your achievements. Are there any that stand out? Now review and reflect, and try to find how best to emulate and use these five skills in your life.

1.

2.

3.

4.

5.

When identifying your skills, keep in mind that a skill doesn't have to be used all the time or used exclusively. You may be good at something that you don't use very often. Remember: Knowledge, or having information about something is not the same as being able to implement—that's the skill. That is, just because you can explain how to drive a car, it doesn't mean you can actually drive it.

Setting unrealistic goals has a sub-context: It's also a form of self-sabotage. Let's use the example of someone like Bob who has a personal goal of having a fulfilling romantic relationship. Nothing wrong with that. The problem is in how: Bob plans on going to a local bar where he hopes to meet the perfect mate, but he only plans on going to the bar one night, and expects to be married within the year. Thinking it through, Bob decides that his effort is futile, and resigns, preferring to "just stay home." In his confused and desperate state, Bob calls up an old flame to see if she'll go out with him. The immediate problem of having someone to date is solved, but Bob may become depressed again when he faces the cold fact that this woman is not a possible long-term partner and that he's very much alone.

A more realistic strategy is for Bob to go to a local bar/bowling alley/gym/golf course and meet one new person and have a good time—not place an unrealistic objective to meet someone and marry in one evening. The new person may not be Ms. Right, but being social without the pressure to meet the right woman is a step in the right direction. Each new person Bob meets opens up new worlds of possibilities. Any one of them could be the person who'll introduce him to the woman he'll marry. In any event, Bob would've had an enjoyable evening rather than feeling despair.

Another kind of unrealistic goal is one you set for someone else. The goal: "I'm going to get my spouse to stop drinking and exercise more," may be noble, but other people, no matter how close, are not obliged to follow your direction. Such aims will only invite frustration and resentment. Similarly, the goal: "I want my spouse to stop criticizing me," is not one you have under your control. You can improve your responses to a spouse's criticism or find a way to defuse it or change it. This does not mean, by the way, that you need to blame yourself or even agree with the criticism, just that you take responsibility for the way you react to it.

There are more realistic goals concerning spouses and improving a marriage. You might say, "I'm going to spend at least 30 minutes more a day talking to my wife/husband," or "I'm going to make sure I say one more encouraging thing to my wife/husband every day." If it's weight control or fitness you want to aim at, try a goal like: "I'm going to make time to exercise three times a week, and invite my spouse to join me."

An Effective Goal Is Rewarding

A target that's too easily reached barely qualifies as a goal in the first place. This is a true rule of thumb, so try not to underestimate yourself and what you can do. Second, if you set a goal that's too easy to reach, you stand the chance of losing interest in pursuing it—as you might with any conquest that seems too easy.

A challenging and more difficult goal requires you to marshal your energy, resources, skills, and focus. It requires a higher level of performance than you may have imagined you had in you. It gives you a higher occasion to rise to, as well as a gratifying way to stretch your capabilities. This *stretch* is a key step to goal setting.

Fortune magazine referred to "stretch goals," as you might suspect, as goals which force you to extend beyond your assumed limits. The term was coined by Jack Welch, former CEO of General Electric, who said of the practice: "*Stretch* means that we try for huge gain while having no idea how to get there—but our people figure out ways to get there." He offered the example of a new VCR built by Toshiba a few years back. The goal had been for GE to produce a comparable VCR with half of the usual parts, in half the time, at half the cost. The team they assigned to the project ended up producing a new model with 60 percent fewer parts in one year instead of the usual two.

Another way to describe "stretch goals" is "extreme goals." The advantage to setting such high and daring goals is that they tend to change and expand your whole sense of what is possible. In the Toshiba example, it might have seemed drastic to try halving the number of parts. But once technicians chased that dream, they realized, why not go further? Why not think bigger? Once you open the floodgates of your potential, prepare to be surprised by what you find. Another name for extreme goals is "Big Hairy Audacious Goals," or BHAGs, a phrase borrowed from authors James Collins and Jerry Porras. In their study of visionary companies, *Built to Last,* these two authors noticed that all 18 companies they profiled shared a similar strategy: They set bold mission statements, which the authors called Big Hairy Audacious Goals. Companies like Disney, Boeing, IBM, and Procter & Gamble, among others, were all pioneers in their fields, and have made permanent changes in the way Americans live, if not people worldwide. Beyond reaching these BHAGs, the companies were profitable, collectively outperforming the stock market fifteen-fold.

So, how exactly can a BHAG make things work? Collins and Porras use the example of America's moon mission in the '60s. President Kennedy and his advisors could have come up with the general goal of, "Let's beef up the space program," left it at that, and been content with small gains. Instead, Kennedy, quite against the conventional wisdom of the day, proclaimed in 1961, that: "This nation should commit itself to achieving the goal, before this decade is out, of landing a man on the moon and returning him safely to earth." His bold confidence inspired Congress to put in $549 million, followed by billions more in subsequent years.

A good BHAG, like Kennedy's statement, should have the following characteristics:

▸ It should be *clear and compelling.* There's no glory in putting it all on the line for a fuzzy and uninteresting "something or other."

▸ It should *engage* people. Reach out and grab them in the gut.

▸ It should also be highly focused, specific, and free from being *"subject to interpretation."*

▸ People should "get it" right away.

Another example: In the late '50s, a small Japanese company, Tokyo Tsushin Kogyo, largely unknown outside of Japan, took the costly step of discarding its old name in favor of a new one: The Sony Corporation. When the company's bank vehemently objected to the idea, Sony's CEO Akio Morita, responded by insisting on the new name. His argument: "Sony" would enable the company to expand worldwide because the name was universally pronounceable. He had big plans for this little company.

Speaking about it later, Morita articulated a vision that transcended merely making a profit: "It became obvious to me that if we did not set our sights on marketing abroad we would not grow into the kind of company that I envisioned. We wanted to change the image around the world of Japanese products being poor in quality."

You need more than a Big Hairy Audacious Goal to be successful, but the advantage of such a goal is that it stimulates progress and effort for a long time. Once one BHAG is reached, it seems more possible to set and reach another BHAG and attain heights never before imagined. Warning: If you do decide to set a BHAG, remember that it should be only a very small part of your overall set of life goals.

An Effective Goal is Tactical, Strategic, and Disciplined

Tactics and strategies are fundamental to the mechanics of reaching a goal. You need effort, persistence, and direction to prevail, and one will not work without the others. Effort is simply trying your best or making a serious attempt to move toward your goals. Persistence is maintaining the course even when the going gets tough. And finally, direction is the course you set to reach your objective. Effort without persistence is too short-lived, and effort without direction is mere activity or busywork. Persistence without direction will get you stuck in a stubborn rut leading nowhere in particular. And just having direction without persistently expending any effort dooms you to live, linger, and get stuck in the domain of dreams. Strategy is a plan of action. It's what you need when your usual way of doing things does not work or when what you're trying to accomplish falls in unfamiliar territory. It is a plan of action that attempts to take all of the variables into account. Strategizing involves conscious problem-solving and creative innovation, rather than the mere execution of learned habits.

The good news is that when you're committed to a goal, many of your skills and behaviors can be marshaled to help you map out strategies. It can even be automatic. To illustrate this point, psychologists like to use the relatively mundane example of reaching a goal such as going grocery shopping. Once you decide to do it, you automatically make a mental or written list, get your wallet, and if you need to, start the car and drive to the store. The act requires no complicated planning or problem solving. Strategy enters into the equation only if your car breaks down or the store closes as you reach the door. Now you strategize by rethinking your plan to get what you need elsewhere.

It takes two seemingly contradictory attitudes to reach a goal: *Seriousness and Flexibility*. Actually, they are key parts of the whole.

Seriousness

You must be serious about striving to reach a goal. Being serious motivates you to take the necessary steps. So what does "being serious" involve, exactly? Basically, it means that you take goal planning to heart and come up with a *strategy*. Goal-planning is all about doing your research, plotting your course, making a step-by-step plan with deadlines, setting short-term and long-term goals, and putting your goals into an estimated overall time frame. Being serious means that if you want to lose weight, you need to research different diets for their healthfulness and effectiveness. If you want to become a talk-show host, you research how other talk-show hosts broke into broadcasting and how they manage their careers.

How can you assure yourself that you're "serious" about your goal? For starters, try writing it down. This shows a certain amount of seriousness in your intention and commitment. The next step: announce your goal publicly. Once you do this, you show a willingness to make your goal something you live up to or face the consequence of a certain amount of embarrassment if it turns out to be more talk than action. Tell people close to you about your goal and take it out of the realm of dreaming and into a destination. Eventually, you'll be able chart the seriousness of your intention by showcasing your achievements.

However, a serious goal is not conditional.

When I hear people couch their aspirations in what I call, "If/then statements," I immediately question the seriousness of their intent. Examples of this include: "If I stay in my current position for just five years, then I'll make enough money to quit and start pursuing my real goals in life full time." Or: "If I wait until after the holidays, then I can start getting in shape." The problem with these statements is that they don't provide momentum or motivation for long-term goals, but on the contrary, they allow momentum to fizzle out. Postponing the pursuit of a goal makes it seem less serious, less urgently desired.

You may not be able to reach a goal right away, but you can begin taking serious steps toward it. Do not bide your time waiting for the right moment to hit. Patience is important, but don't be so "patient" that you sit back and wait for a sign that the perfect conditions are opening up, which after all, may never occur.

The poet/novelist Charles Bukowski wrote a poem about this very syndrome entitled, "Light and Space and Time." In it, an artist boasts about how he has finally quit his job and can afford a studio with enough space and light to paint. The artist had always been sure that with these things finally in place, he could become a real painter. Bukowski, who wrote his many books under all sorts of less-than-perfect circumstances, implies that "light and space and time" have little to do with the creation of art. A true artist will create, no matter what the conditions.

So, if you want to write a novel, don't say, "If I ever find time with my busy schedule, then I'll write that novel." This suggests that your need to write a novel is probably less important than continuing on your busy schedule. The novel is more of a dream, than something you can make real for yourself. Rather, if you really want to do it, start writing wherever you can, whenever you can, grabbing up whatever available minutes before, or after, your work day. You may be able to complete your version of a 300-page masterpiece line-by-line and page-by-page, although it will take you longer than if you had had concentrated time. This way, you can get on your way, building momentum toward reaching your goal of finishing a novel. Hundreds of published writers have written books around their "real jobs," putting down sentence after sentence until the book is done. This includes author Mario Puzo, who wrote *The Godfather* while holding down a full-time magazine job to support his family.

Writing It Down

It's not enough to have an idea of where you're going. Give your ideas and goals words, and an image to hold onto. Writing down your goals shows that you're making a minimal commitment to them, making them real and important. Writing down your goals is the first step to making them happen. Keep in mind, many of you will be uncomfortable writing your goals down for the very reason you should be writing them down—

the fear of your goals becoming clearer. Let me explain—as you have a clearer picture of your direction, it becomes more real, thus creating discomfort. The discomfort comes from seeing how difficult it might be or how long it might take to reach your objective—it can be overwhelming. Don't let this discomfort intimidate you—keep your focus.

The power of writing down goals was famously illustrated in a study conducted at Yale University in 1953. Researchers asked students if they had specific written goals and a plan for achieving them. Only three percent had such written goals. Twenty years later, the researchers interviewed all of the surviving members of the class of 1953. They found that the three percent with specific, recorded goals were worth more financially than the other 97 percent all put together. Financial worth does not tell the whole story, but there were other indications that the three percent were also more content and happy with their lives on the whole than were their classmates.

So given the overwhelming evidence of its usefulness, why doesn't everyone write their goals down? Psychologists Edwin Locke and Gary Platham, who have done extensive research on goal-setting theory and behavior, note that goal setting may cause anxiety for some people. A goal can be seen as a threat; it suggests standards of performance that must be met. It suggests a disconnection between reality and desire. It carries the possibility of failure, or not measuring up to your own expectations.

People who fear failure hesitate to put themselves in any situation that causes them discomfort. Many stop setting goals altogether, falling into a pattern of underachievement. My hope is that if you learn nothing else from this book, you will at least stop fearing failure and see it for what it is—a necessary learning experience rather than a permanent stamp. (Reread Chapter 3 on Failure to understand how "failing" can really be a positive learning experience.)

Flexibility

Being flexible and receptive to feedback only strengthens your quest to reach your goals with serious and single-minded dedication. Interestingly, seriousness and flexibility are not opposites here, but counterparts in a bigger plan. Flexibility is just as important as seriousness and focus. To ensure that you're being as flexible as necessary, you must integrate three components into your goal-planning regimen: *adaptability and overcoming obstacles, reassessment,* and *feedback.*

Adaptability and Overcoming Obstacles—
Coming Up with "Plan B"

Although this Chapter maps out strategies to help you meet your personal goals, it's important to remember that sometimes, even the best-laid plans go awry. When life throws you a curve ball, you're forced to adjust both your expectations and your goals. It happens all the time.

I'll give you an example from my own life: I planned a hiking expedition with my friend Steven and envisioned a brisk hike in the mountains. My goals were to relax, get in touch with nature, reflect, and bond with my friend. What I did not know was that Steven, an avid rock-climber, was planning to take us straight up the mountain. We started hiking on the trail, came to a rock face, and started to climb. I thought the rock face led to the rest of the hiking trial—I was wrong. After climbing for about 15 minutes, I asked Steven when we would get back to the trail. That's when he explained. I looked back to where we had started, saw a huge drop, and realized there was no going back—our hiking trail had turned into a serious rock face. The top of the rock was still a good 300 yards away. I breathed deeply and tried to focus, and promptly forgot all about getting in touch with nature, reflecting on my life, relaxing, yadda, yadda, yadda. My new goal was to get to the top of that rock in one piece, and the only way to do that was one step at a time. I concentrated intently on each hand and foot placement and slowly made my way up the face of the mountain.

When I reached the top, I looked back down and gasped in amazement. My first thought was, "That was so stupid! I could have been killed doing that!" My second thought was to never speak to my friend again, but my third thought was, "Wow! I can't believe I climbed that thing!" When I really needed to, I was able to shift my priorities to match my changed circumstances. I don't intend to become a rock climber, but it was good to know I could make this shift when I needed to.

While adaptability helps you troubleshoot any anticipated or unanticipated obstacles, once you identify an obstacle, you can chart alternate paths to your goal. Say, for example, that your goal is to be head of the company you work for in ten years. Think of what obstacles might stand in your way. You need to come up with a Plan B for overcoming these potential obstacles or setbacks.

The current head of the company may remain in his position if the company is successful. Someone might be brought in from outside. Perhaps a coworker will compete with you for the job. How do you compete to outshine that person? How will you react? What will be your alternate path? You could get a job at another company where the prospects for climbing the ladder are better. What company? Be specific.

Could you start your own company? This is not something you can do impulsively. What kind of company would you want to own? Be specific. How would you start it? Who would you enlist to help you with it? How would you make a business plan and get funding? Setting up and thinking through these alternate paths on paper is not a simple task. Take time with it. Set yourself a deadline of two weeks to reflect on your ideas. One of the advantages in this strategy is that you emerge feeling you have a variety of options rather than being stuck with all your eggs in a single basket. Such a feeling also gives you leverage and confidence.

While you're developing your goal-planning strategy, you're likely to encounter moments of uncertainty about what to do next. Earmark these gaps of uncertainty for special study. For instance, your career plan may require you to go back to school, but you're not sure yet how you'll pay for further study. Make a note to yourself that you'll need to investigate financial aid and how to get low-cost student loans.

Another example: If your goal is to lose 20 pounds, and your efforts up until now have been unsuccessful, seek out help. You may need to consult an expert such as a personal trainer, nutritionist, or even a psychologist specializing in weight-loss issues.

To go after what you really want, you must take risks. Goal planning doesn't completely eliminate risks, but it does help you to take the right risks, at the right times. It also can minimize crises by helping you visualize obstacles and how you will prevail over them.

Reassessing Your Situation

When you're on the path toward a goal, you need to constantly reassess where you've been and where you're going. You can develop the most thorough plan and strategize until the end of time, but reality and new information still will intrude, and you'll have to adapt. There are, in all likelihood, a variety of ways to reassess.

First, *make a periodic assessment of where you stand in relation to your goal.* This should take the shape of a chart that marks your progress—check off the steps you've taken and keep track of the ones still to come. Many people find that keeping a daily journal or diary is tremendously useful. Your plan will require frequent tweaking, sometimes demanding a complete revision. Put yourself on a schedule of monthly assessments, or aim for every three or six months depending on the time frame.

Don't go overboard with your assessment. Unless you're an extremely detail-oriented person, don't try and make daily plans to reassess. This becomes too obsessive and can lead you into a forest of details that obscures the larger picture. Some studies show that overly specific plans can be counterproductive. This certainly rings true in your business and personal lives. Imagine how unhealthy it would be if, for example, it were your goal to meet and marry someone, and you assessed your romantic relationship on a daily basis. This would leave little room for spontaneity or for a genuine love to grow.

Daily over-structured plans restrict the room for choice, discretion, and creativity, and this rigidity can be oppressive, taking all the joy out of striving. Making choices is part of the pleasure of striving and keeps you engaged in the process. In addition, daily planning may take more time away from the actual work of achieving your goals. Finally, overly specific plans tend to breed more experiences of failure and frustration, experiences which may emotionally deflate you and cause you to lose momentum.

All that said, it doesn't mean you can't break things down into daily requirements to meet your goals—or "tasks to completion" lists. As a consultant and a manager to corporations, I have often suggested creating daily goal requirements to meet overall goals. For example, an objective like having a new accounts manual within four weeks, at first may seem daunting, but when we planned out and broke down goals by the day, it became a manageable project.

Remember, don't try planning techniques that are overly complicated that you won't stick to—all you'll be doing is sabotaging your goals. You can start out by planning once a year if you think you will have trouble keeping up, and over time you can develop more sophisticated goal planning techniques.

Seek and Be Receptive to Feedback

Feedback from other people is important because no matter how thorough you've been in your research and planning, you may have overlooked an important aspect of reaching the goal. You can also lose perspective or the ability to accurately judge the quality of your own efforts, something you regain with the help of wise and thoughtful friends and advisers.

Being receptive to feedback from others also reduces the risk of boredom and relieves some of the inherent feelings of loneliness when in pursuit of a goal. One study found that schoolchildren preferred computer games that offered a clear goal and feedback about performance. The same principle applies to sports, where score keeping lets each team know where it stands.

Weight loss also provides a good example. It helps to get on the scale every once in a while, but climbing on every day gives an inaccurate reading of weight-loss progress because there are hour-to-hour variations in body weight. In the same vein, a "reading" of feedback on your goals is subject to similar, if precarious, fluctuations. You may expect too much too soon and judge the true state of your progress too quickly. Another example is saving and investing money. If you watch the stock market everyday you will have unrealistic views; it's more important to look at yearly returns. Reasonably spaced quantitative feedback lets you know where you stand in relation to a goal. It will also let you know when you need to redouble your efforts or even come up with a whole new game plan.

Remember: Don't use feedback as an excuse not to meet your goals. If you acquire inaccurate feedback, it can be a substantial demotivator. Start-up businesses often convene a board of advisers who are experts in the field. You can do the same in the business of life, that is, assemble your own "board." Choose people who you turn to for advice and who can aid and guide you appropriately. Your "board" should be concerned about your well-being, not have hidden agendas, and if possible, one or two board members should demonstrate knowledge in the area of your interest. If your goal is to open a restaurant, seek the advice of restaurateurs or chefs you admire; in addition, survey friends and associates whose taste you respect. If two or more people on your board whose opinions you respect tell you that you're way off base, then it's worthwhile to hear them out and ask for advice.

Here, too, when it comes to getting feedback, seek a balance. At certain times, you need to put your head down, charge forward, and go alone without outside interference or help. And if you've really done your research and homework, you will have faith in your expertise. For instance, let's say you want to write a novel. Ill-timed negative feedback could be devastatingly discouraging at too early a stage, and could ultimately lead you to abandon your efforts.

Don't Give In to Ego Threats

We all know how it feels to have someone threaten our ego even in seemingly innocuous ways. If you've ever played golf or another sport with friends, you know what it's like to step up to the tee and hear someone say, "You'll never reach that green in one shot." Comments like this, widely used to psych out an opponent in sports, get your adrenaline pumping, your hands sweating, and affect your game. You may blast the ball to kingdom come to prove your friend wrong, and end up shanking it, overshooting it, or watching your perfect shot drop like a stone in the lake. Instead of hitting the best shot you can, you aim for the best shot in history, and thereby do worse than you would have had you stuck to your game plan. If you substitute the hole-in-one with your goal, you can see how such a response is self-sabotaging—a misdirected surrender to an "ego threat."

What are they?

Even people with high self-esteem are susceptible to what psychologists call "ego threats." You're apt to suffer an ego threat when people you care about voice doubts about your ability to achieve the goals you say you will. The fact is that you trust these people, and their undermining sentiments hurt you. Ego threats come from a variety of sources, but the most powerful come from the people closest to you. That's why they're so dangerous: They come from people you want to impress. Parents are infamous for posing ego threats: "You'll never amount to anything," or the seemingly less brutal, "You're too picky about boy/girlfriends. You have to lower your standards or you'll be single your whole life." As a response to these threats, you might tell yourself, "Well, someday, I'm going to be the President of the United States," or "I'm going to marry a supermodel." You can set unreasonably high standards for yourself and lose touch with what's important when you're determined to prove someone wrong.

Or you can use ego threats as an excuse to give up. It's also not unusual to believe the doubt—such as accepting that you'll never amount to much—and rashly change a goal and jeopardize the chances of getting what you want. This makes what others think of your goals more important than what you think of yourself.

Sometimes you may thrive when people tell you what you cannot do. How many people told John F. Kennedy he was crazy for predicting we'd put a man on the moon by the end of the '60s? The desire to prove doubters wrong may provide you with the energy to succeed, but learn to distinguish between doubts and ego threats and don't undermine your own interests.

For example, say you have a goal to write a novel this year. A friend says, "You can't write a novel—it takes amazing discipline and great writing skills. I know you. You don't have the patience." This could spur you to work harder and *prove to yourself you have what it takes.* The mere presence of a doubt does not make the goal unreachable. But if you respond by trying to write an entire book in one sitting, you've altered your goal and made a bad plan that is bound to fail.

Goals in the Context of the Rest of Your Life

You don't live in a vacuum. Your actions and decisions affect your loved ones to one degree or another. Even those of you who are single have family, coworkers, and friends who are affected by your actions. So, when setting a goal, you need to take these relationships into account by asking questions such as:

▸ How does this goal affect my family?

▸ How does this goal affect my responsibilities at work?

▸ How does this goal affect my friends and coworkers?

▸ How does this goal relate to the other activities in my life?

▸ Will I need to give up some activities to make room for it?

▸ How does it relate to my community or environment?

If you sense that you're encountering friction from others in pursuit of your goal, you need to confront this issue head-on before proceeding. Discuss your goals with your loved ones. More than likely, they'll be pleased that you've decided to make a positive change. If they have any worries, you can assure them that you know what you're doing. For example, let's say you're married and decide to train for an upcoming marathon. In all likelihood, your spouse will be thrilled for you and happy to see you in great physical shape. But he or she might also be concerned that such training will take away from some valuable family time. To take such concerns into account, perhaps your spouse will opt to do some of the training with you, or you could offer to cut down on other things, like watching TV or working at the office, and use that time to train.

Summing Up

▸ Reaching a goal requires effort, persistence, and direction and you need all three to prevail. Effort without persistence is too short-lived, and effort without direction is mere activity or busywork. Persistence without direction will get you stuck in a stubborn rut leading nowhere.

▸ A goal doesn't have to be something extraordinary—don't be intimidated into thinking you must have a perceived dynamic goal. You can simply want to create a family or buy a new car every two years or get a promotion at work.

▸ Stick with one goal at a time and make it a sound, quality goal. Setting more than one goal can dilute your efforts and provide you with an excuse for failing to reach any goal.

▸ Goal planning is not meant to eliminate risks. Taking risks is essential to go after what you really want and planning helps you to take the right risks at the right time.

▸ You can minimize crises by anticipating obstacles and planning for how you will surmount them.

▸ Don't set goals with a false sense of optimism that everything will go smoothly and right the first time. You may be so disappointed that you'll be tempted to dismiss the goal as unreachable.

▸ Discipline is a continuous experience. It means staying on track toward your dreams. A vision of your future keeps you motivated, but discipline directs you down the path.

CHAPTER SIX

If You Can See "It" . . . "It" Can Happen

You have to expect things of yourself before
you can do them.
—Michael Jordan

I can't imagine that everyone doesn't practice
visualization whether they are aware of it or not.
I can tell you for a fact, and I've talked to enough writers,
that virtually every writer sits at the word processor at some point
and imagines the reviews of the book, or how the book is going to look,
or winning awards for the book. I think these are the kinds of things
that get you through the process.
—Neal Gabler, author of *An Empire of Their Own*

Visualization is another way of saying that your goal is a "view of the future." Many people have found it tremendously helpful and motivational to imagine the feelings and positive rewards that come with the achievement of goals. Others aren't sure how to imagine a goal and how to capture the feelings. I've devoted the majority of this chapter to a technique that works for anyone who wants to use it—athletes, business people, smokers, overweight individuals, artists, and problem solvers. It's called "visualization" and it works. The second part of this chapter focuses on the use of visualization and the information learned in the first part of Goals to create a very specific goal-planning chart. *Remember, it is an act of self-love and self-affirmation to visualize yourself in a better and happier place.*

Visualization

Let's say that your dream is to start what will become a very successful business. While this is a worthy and even fairly common goal, it is, of course, not an easy thing to accomplish. The rewards of turning a profit may be a long way away with many intermediate steps of developing a business plan, getting financing, finding a location, and more. One way to keep the faith in the midst of exhausting hard work is to hone your skills at visualizing the outcome—and to *keep this vision close at hand* to summon when the going gets rough. When you can "see" an appealing image of an attainable future, it informs and inspires your actions, and helps to coordinate your plan and goals. At the same time, you should not live entirely in the future. You need to visualize and create step-by-step smaller goals along the way.

Why is developing this visual image so critical to your success down the line?

Well, think of achieving goals as a long road trip—for instance, a road trip to Saskatchewan. At first, Saskatchewan might sound like just a cold, distant place—or at the very least, just a *really* long drive. But say someone showed you where it is on the map, and told you that your destination was in a beautiful area of north central Canada that you'd always wanted to visit—then you might be more interested in the trip. Then maybe he or she would show you a brochure on what was waiting for you there—the adorable bed and breakfast by the lake where you'd be staying; menus and photos from some of the local restaurants featuring locally harvested fresh vegetables and salmon; scenic vistas and beautiful mountain walks; an exhibit that would interest you at one of the nearby museums. As you see these images vividly, the drive is starting to seem a little more doable now, isn't it?

Now, that same someone takes out a map and shows you the route north, including some scenic stops along the way, and other pleasant side trips you can take while you're on the road. All of the sudden, the trip doesn't sound so insurmountable—you might enjoy the drive itself, and even during the long, boring stretches, you could be entertained by the thought of what's waiting for you. This is the power of visualization. It helps you to create the road map, stay on course, and reach your destination.

What Is Visualization All About?

You hear the word "visualization" a lot these days but what does it mean, and how can it help you? Practicing visualization can help you break out of a rut, or break through an obstacle, much as a martial arts expert shatters boards, that appears "unbreakable." It can raise your expectations about your life and what you'd like to achieve, help you define your goals, then motivate you to reach them. If you have no specific goal in mind yet, visualization can set into motion the process of finding your goals.

Everyone visualizes, but children are the group to watch here. When they talk about what they want to be when they "grow-up," they delve into their fantasy world. They talk about the dream, read about it, dress up like what they want to be, and constantly imagine themselves in that role. Allow yourself this important childlike gift. You still have it.

In fact, film directors have been using this process since the beginning of the movie-making industry—they call it storyboarding. This is the process of illustrating every single shot in the entire film, detailing exactly how it will be shot, the actors' expressions, and many other specifics.

Visualization can begin with something as a simple as a daydream, a fantasy—a free-floating ride through the tangles of your imagination.

You've no doubt heard that fantasizing can improve your sex life. Well, it can improve the rest of your life as well. Perhaps you have learned to censor your imagination, thinking you should not be frittering away valuable time with mere daydreams. But this is *daydreaming with a purpose.* You are exploring who you are, and getting to know your aspirations and desires. By the way, daydreaming without a purpose is not so bad either and can provide you with information about yourself.

The next phase addresses the kind of visualization that has a very specific goal in mind, which is an essential part of achievement. Let me tell you a story about how this kind of visualization helped me. For a long time, I struggled with the fact that I wanted to be in better physical shape. But I went about it all wrong. I exercised without following a diet correctly, or sometimes followed a diet without getting the necessary exercise. Although the information about how to lose weight and get in better shape certainly was readily available in local bookstores, and on the Internet, I avoided seeking it out. *That was my pattern.* For 35 years, I was a master at making "efforts to avoid efforts." Why was I engaging in such self-sabotage? Some essential piece was missing. I had not and could not visualize a new physical image of myself. My sense of possibility was limited by the reality of what I saw in the mirror. I had no idea where I was going, and what to aim for.

Finally, I broke through. I began to visualize myself in optimum physical shape and health. It was more than just an image; I also could "see" and understand how it would feel to be in the physical shape I'd always wanted to be in. It was the supreme "Aha!" moment because, not only could I perfectly envision a new, slimmed down, more attractive version of myself, I could also envision the path to that goal. From there, the goal planning and discipline fell into place because the benefits were completely apparent to me. The rewards were no longer vague and empty phrases, such as "looking better" or "feeling more attractive." Visual imagery made the benefits tangible to me, and motivation ceased to be a problem. Whenever I was discouraged and lost enthusiasm, I remembered the thoughts and feelings from my visualization of achieving my goals. I also used visualization to create a plan of action to achieve my goals. I thought through how I was going to exercise each day, prepare my own foods, and what I was going to do when I had an insatiable craving. I also mentally rehearsed what I was going to say at restaurants or to friends when asked about my "strange" eating habits.

People who have seen me since I have shaved off much of my excess weight, and kept it off, cannot get over the change. My slim self looks very different from my overweight self. To say it's worthwhile looking for that person on the inside, then making it happen on the outside is an understatement. I'm living proof that visualization works.

When you're stuck in a bad pattern, part of the reason can be a *failure of vision*. You're not seeing clearly so you cannot see your way out of a predicament. You're not seeing what lies beneath the surface or the painful feelings that drive you to your addictions, shortcomings or self-sabotaging patterns. Most likely, you're acting and reacting blindly and automatically. To break out of a negative pattern, visualize where you want to go and what it will feel like to be free of this particular shackle. It will clear your sight, so to speak.

When trying to break yourself of negative thoughts or patterns, imagine yourself without that pattern or without those thoughts. You can use visualization techniques to accomplish this.

Visualization In Action

Weight loss and fitness are a very worthwhile goals, but visualization has been applied to goals far more sublime. Albert Einstein wrote that, "Imagination is more important than knowledge." He told the story of how he used thought experimentation to visualize what the world would look like if one traveled at the speed of light. These imaginative leaps eventually led to his theory of spatial relativity. Of course, there was much hard work, perseverance, and many steps in between. But the journey would not have been possible without that first step.

Michelangelo also used a kind of visualization, what he called *intelleto*. The great artist believed that the form he sought in a block of marble already existed in the stone and he was just the means by which the true form of the stone could emerge. To see that true or ideal form, he needed "*intelleto*"—the capacity to see things as they truly are or are meant to be, which is also a kind of imagination. Imagination, not some hard-nosed realism, is the starting point for many great achievements.

Athletes, too, are master practitioners of visualization. They have to be to succeed. World record-setting decathlete Dan O'Brien was the heavy favorite to win the gold medal at the 1992 Olympics in Seoul. He was on his way to the gold when the inconceivable happened—he failed to qualify in the pole vault. Since he was so far ahead in the other events, he was allowed to compete in the pole vault competition as well. But he failed to clear the bar on all three attempts. He would have to wait another four years to try and win the title in Atlanta in 1996. In the years between, O'Brien rejected the idea of consulting a sports psychologist, but he worked on himself mentally while continuing his physical training. "Milt Campbell, the 1956 gold medallist and the first black man to win a decathlon, told me that it takes place in your mind first," said O'Brien in an interview in the months leading up to the 1996 games. "If I don't wake up every day thinking I'm going to win the Olympic gold medal, I won't." When Dan O'Brien captured gold in Atlanta, he had already envisioned his victory many times.

Another example of visualization being used to improve an athlete's objectives was during the 2000 Olympic games in Sydney when 16-year-old Megan Quann upset the defending Olympic champion, Penny Heyns of South Africa, in the 100-meter breaststroke. Quann had promised at the American Olympic trials that Heyns was "going down." Quann had imagined victory as she had every night before the event, taking a stop-watch to bed and visualizing her race stroke by stroke. "I can see the tiles at the bottom of the pool, I can hear the crowd cheering, I can taste the water," Quann said of her ritual.

One reason that visualization is so essential is because it infuses you with a sense of self-confidence, and makes you feel that your goals are both real and reachable. It gives you energy and desire, and helps maintain motivation. It's understandable that visualization has crossed over from the "New Age" category and has been widely adopted by the world of business. Tom Watson, the founder of IBM, tells this story in Michael E. Gerber's *The E-Myth Revisited* about how IBM's success was first made real in his mind:

> IBM is what it is today for three very special reasons. The first reason is that, at the beginning, I had a clear picture of what the company would look like when I was done. You might say I had a model in my mind of what it would look like when the dream—my vision—was in place.
>
> The second reason was that once I had that picture, I asked myself how a company which looked like that would have to act. I then created a picture of how IBM would act when it was finally done.
>
> The third reason IBM has been so successful was that unless we began to act this way from the very beginning, we would never get there. In other words, I realized that for IBM to become a great company, it would have to act like a great company before it ever became one.
>
> From the very outset, IBM was fashioned after the template of my vision. And each and every day, we

attempted to model the company after the template. At the end of each day, we asked ourselves how well we did, discovered the disparity between where we were and where we had committed ourselves to be, and at the start of the following day set out to make up for the difference.

Every day at IBM was a day devoted to business development, not doing business. We didn't do business at IBM, we built one.

Mental Rehearsal

It was Michael Jordan who said, "Basketball is more mental than physical." A specific type of visualization known as *mental rehearsal* has been proven to increase achievement in sports and other areas of human endeavor. Studies have shown that performance improves with mental practice, just as it does with physical practice.

In a study conducted by the National Institutes of Health, the brain patterns of volunteers were monitored as they each learned a new skill: in this case, a simple five-finger exercise on the piano. One group practiced daily for two hours and another group sat at the piano for two hours, hitting the keys without learning anything. Those in the first group showed tremendous changes in the part of the brain dealing with the use of hand muscles. "They more than tripled the size of their brains' motor maps," said Dr. Alvaro Pascal-Leone, one of the researchers. "And these changes paralleled the improvement in their performance." Volunteers who just tickled the ivories aimlessly showed little or no change in their brain patterns.

But the biggest surprise came from volunteers in a third group who were taught the piano exercise, but were only allowed to rehearse it mentally—*not manually*—while looking at the keyboard. After five days, their brain patterns were identical to the ones who had actually practiced and thought about it, the researchers reported.

Similar studies showing that subjects who mentally rehearse basketball free throws for an hour each day improve their performance nearly or equal to subjects who actually do practice shooting. The reason is that the neural pathways are trained and the muscles in the body "fire" as if a person were actually performing the activity. The amount of actual activity may be scarcely noticeable, but the result—what is called *muscle memory*—is the same as physical practice.

"It definitely enhances learning," says Jean Williams, a sports psychologist at the University of Arizona and former president of the American Association for the Advancement of Applied Sports Psychology. "You can learn new techniques faster than if you just do physical practice, and you can refine performance."

Still other studies have shown that athletes can also recuperate from injury faster by maintaining their timing through systematic visual imaging.

Most of the world's top athletes engage in mental rehearsal before a big event. Six-time Ironman triathlon winner Mark Allen, for example, goes on spiritual retreats as he prepares for the grueling event. He focuses on how he will overcome the pain and trains himself to block it out. World-class skiers imagine each run down the slope, perfectly executing each turn, to "train" their bodies to do the same when they actually compete. Everyone engages in some type of mental rehearsal throughout the day. When you imagine getting home and relaxing after a long hard day, or when you go through in your mind how you're going to respond to your child's bad report card, these are, in a way, forms of mental rehearsal. In these cases, though, it is not exactly a conscious or intentional activity the way it is when a top athlete prepares and calls up the needed images.

Mental rehearsal may also reduce anxiety before and during a performance. Psychologist and former all-American swimmer, Marcia Middel, Ph.D., says she uses these techniques to help athletes and musicians overcome performance anxiety. Basketball Hall-of-Famer Bill Russell, the only man to win a staggering 11 NBA championships, described an experience he had at age 18 while watching a basketball game from the bench:

> Something happened that night that opened my eyes and chilled my spine. I was sitting on the bench watching Treu and McKelvey the way I always did. Every time one of them would make one of the moves I liked, I'd close my eyes just afterward and try to see the play in my mind . . . I'd try to create an instant replay on the inside of my eyelids . . . On this particular night, I was working on replays of many plays including McKelvey's way of taking an offensive rebound and moving to the hoop. It's a fairly simple play for any big man in basketball, but I didn't execute it well and McKelvey did. Since I had an accurate vision of his technique in my head, I started playing with the image right there on the bench, running back the pictures several times and each time inserting a part of me for McKelvey.
>
> Finally, when I saw myself making the whole move, I ran this over and over. When I went in the game, I grabbed an offensive rebound and put it in the basket just the way McKelvey did. It seemed natural, almost as if I were stepping into a film and following the signs. When the imitation worked and the ball went in, I could barely contain myself. I was so elated, I thought I'd float right out of the gym. Now, for the first time I had transferred

something from my head to my body. It seemed so easy.
My first dose of athletic confidence was coming to me
when I was 18 years old.

Mental rehearsal can also be used to help you create a plan of action
and help you stay on track with all the details that develop along the way
to achieving your goals. Sharon, a computer programmer, wanted to become an architect. She realized that it would be a difficult career change,
and would require more education, which means she would have to continue working while she received her degree. She also understood the
hard work and long hours that she had ahead of her. She sat down day
after day, and worked through in her head exactly what it was going to
be like on a typical day, working full-time and studying architecture in
the evenings. She realized the more she went through this process, the
more she learned and understood about her decision. By mentally rehearsing typical days, Sharon knew that she would lose interest in work,
and could get fired. She also became aware that working fewer hours
was crucial because otherwise she wouldn't be able to concentrate on
her classes.

When she finally made the change, she was prepared. Sharon had
found a new job working as a computer programmer in an architecture
firm; she cut her hours but got basically the same pay. Sharon knew what
to expect, and had the mental energy to move forward as a result. By
being mentally prepared she was able to avoid much of the stress, and
many of the tribulations that would have normally occurred when making such a tremendous career change.

How to Start the Visualization Process

You can start the visualization process by allowing your thoughts to
travel wildly and in an unstructured fashion. This is primarily used to get

you started—especially if you're not sure how to visualize or you're having trouble understanding what you want to achieve. The concept is to give yourself the freedom to imagine, and as your objectives become clearer, you can graduate to using visualization as a more defined procedure.

This can take effort if it has been a long time since you have dreamed in this way. Creating visual imagery that you can use for both inspiration and motivation takes practice. You need to program or reprogram your brain to achieve a goal.

Visualization should not be too easy. If it comes entirely without effort, then it may yield only mediocre results. Even in your visualization process, you need to push beyond the obvious limits you've unconsciously set for yourself, and instead, strive for better and better results.

Visualization Step-by-Step

Make time, perhaps a regular time, for visualizing and daydreaming every day. Make it count and build toward some realization by trying to pick up where you left off the day before. Add detail each time—the more detail, the better. At first, don't visualize obstacles and problems you might encounter along the road. Try to see yourself at the goal, the finish line, and then fill in all of the textures—including the possible problems and obstacles.

Visualization is the first essential step. Before figuring out how you'll get to where you want to go, you need to know in detail where you want to be. You have to get comfortable with the notion of yourself as a person who can accomplish your goals.

1. **Sit in a comfortable, quiet place**.

2. **Close your eyes and dream**.

    It may seem fuzzy or disjointed at first. Don't try to force the daydream into some sort of coherent logic yet. Let it drift wildly. See how far you can go.

3. **Concentrate and imagine**.
Concentrate on, and imagine what you would like to do, accomplish, achieve—or simply just let your mind fantasize and wander.

4. **Focus on something a little more specific**.
After letting your mind go out there, reel it back in a bit, and try to focus on something a little more specific. Try to focus on a goal.

It is important that you eventually get very specific with your visualization. Make sure to compose a specific goal, not an overall goal like losing weight, but something more detailed—for example, "My overall goal is to lose ten pounds by January 10, and one of the many ways I need to improve my diet is lunch. I always go out to eat and get caught up in a feeding frenzy, especially when we go to Patsy's for Italian food . . ." Remember: If you find yourself in a visualization process that seems too easy—meaning it lacks some frustration—the process will not prove as effective as when you really put in the effort.

Neuro-Linguistic Programming (NLP), is a technique that has been developed to help people focus visual imagery. The key to NLP is to control what are called sub-modalities. These are the variations that occur in our dreams where, for example, the colors may be bright, faded, or in black and white.

When you visualize goals, you want them to be bright and distinct. You want the sounds to be cheerful. You want the feeling to be comfortable and upbeat. If your visual images appear faded and unfocused, you want to make them brighter and clearer. If you imagine how others would see you, you want to change your vision so you are inside yourself and can feel how it is to be there.

This type of distinct visualization can be called "dreaming in color." In his book, *Dreaming In Technicolor: A Rehearsal for Success,* writer Sydney Friedman tells the story of a teenager named Freddie who lived in his neighborhood. Freddie was so anxious to get his driver's license that he became obsessed with the idea of driving. He would make excuses to ride in any car, anytime, with anybody. He would sit next to the driver and steer an imaginary steering wheel. He would stomp on imaginary pedals. As soon as he was eligible, he rushed down to driving school to take his first class. The instructor said, "start the car," and Freddie drove off like a pro. He was so good, the instructor accused him of having driven illegally. Freddie hadn't done any such thing. He just knew how to visualize in color.

If you have trouble getting started or getting around to creating visualizations that you know would be valuable for you to do, try the following:

▸ Pause to ask yourself if there are any genuine objections in your mind to completing this task. Be sensitive to them. If there are no major obstacles, continue.

▸ Think about the end result of getting this task done. Imagine how you will gain in many ways from getting this done.

▸ Now use your imagination, all of your senses, to change how you think about getting the job done. Make the images of the benefits bigger, closer, more colorful, etc. Add pleasant sounds, an encouraging voice, or whatever will make the experience more attractive to you. Keep doing this until you feel strongly attracted to the task itself.

In the end, your visualization should be so clear that there will be no doubt that what you are working for is what you really want.

5. **Think about what it will be like to have achieved that goal.**
Give this a great deal of thought and detail, and include sounds, smells, feelings, and tastes. Make the image colorful, detailed, rich, and vibrant. Start to fill out some of the contours of your daydream. What does it look and feel like? What would it be like to live in the world that you are conjuring up for yourself. What kind of people will be there? How will they act? How will you interact with them? Get a clear idea or picture of it.

Make sure you use all of your senses. Focused visualization in practice entails more than just using your sense of vision, both internal and external. NLP emphasizes this. In the book, *NLP: The New Technology of Achievement,* I found an example of how this works:

A man wanted to eat better, but he couldn't summon the willpower to choose an apple over a piece of chocolate cake when it came time for a snack. He decided to use visualization to imagine how his mind perceived different types of foods. He found that chocolate cake, for example, was very vivid and richly detailed in his imagination, spongy, sweet smelling, and mouth-wateringly tasty. On the other hand, when he imagined apples and other vegetables and fruits, they were black and white, with only vague textures and smells and virtually no taste. So, he took it upon himself to change the sub-modalities of his vision. He made the chocolate cake and other sweets less attractive in his mind by making them flat, black and white and more distant. Then he worked on envisioning fruits and vegetables in 3-D Technicolor, fresh-smelling, crunchy, and savory. This revisioning had an immediate impact on his eating habits, and he started choosing healthier foods because they had become more attractive in his mind.

If you don't know anything about the world you are fantasizing, you can begin to do research on it. If your dream is to be a corporate executive or a social worker, try to find out something about those worlds so that you can visualize them more clearly. Make your daydream as convincing to yourself as possible. For inspiration, check out the biography section of your local bookstore and read about people who had similar goals and desires as yours, and learn how they think, things they've done, how they react to setbacks and reinvent themselves.

When visualizing, it's important to let yourself go—to spend time thinking about what it would be like to live in and be a part of the world that you dream of. So if you want to be a firefighter, computer programmer, or anything else, you should "walk the walk" and "talk the talk." Get more information about what you want and read about the subject, go to lectures, join clubs, subscribe to magazines (on the subject), and surround yourself with people with the same interest or profession.

When I decided I wanted to write films, the first thing I did was learn everything there was about screen writing. I'd go to cafés where I knew other screenwriters worked or hung out. I befriended many of them and as a result, learned the trade to a certain degree.

6. **Visualize the steps it will take to achieve that goal, then visualize yourself successfully taking those steps**.

Think of yourself as a director of a movie that is about your own life. You choose and control the images, the story, the soundtrack, the costumes, and the textures.

If you want to lose weight, imagine what you will look like when you attain your goal. Now, move beyond the external vision of yourself and put yourself inside this new you. What kind of clothes will you be able to wear as a result? Will looking fitter impact on your career or social life? Think of how great it will feel to be in great shape.

In fact, one of the training exercises that I use in counseling weight-loss clients is to have them come up with three different visualizations of success. Each client is asked to write down three different circumstances or "Life Preservers" of what it would be like when she reaches her goal weight.

For example, one client, Samantha, wrote about running into her first husband who used to mock her weight problem. She describes, "I was exhausted, but I had just come from an art opening, and was stepping out of a cab—that's when he saw me. He gasped, almost in shock at how much weight I'd lost—and how good I looked . . ." Samantha created three of these very detailed visualizations, and was asked to use these as motivational tools anytime she ran into a "food crisis." Any time she's tempted to go off of her weight-loss program she would think about one of her visualizations or "Life Preservers," and use it as a motivator to fend off her craving.

Let yourself lose control of "the movie" every once in while, and see where it takes you. Remember, you are the director. If you don't like where the story is going, you can rewind, recut, and revise the script.

7. **Get further into the details**.

Break these details down into imaginary steps. Think and write down your own view of how you would act and behave in order to move toward this very targeted goal. Be specific and go into the nitty-gritty details—don't spare a thought.

Give a step-by-step description of exactly what your experience would be like. For example:

We normally go to Patsy's on Tuesdays and Thursdays. I'm going to pick up the phone (tomorrow morning before work) and call Patsy's and request a low-fat, low-calorie meal in advance . . . I'll ask for some grilled fish or poultry with no oil or butter. I'll tell them I'm embarrassed to ask in person, to have it ready every Tuesday and Thursday, and I will call in the morning to make sure they know.

Next, I'm imagining myself getting in the car to go to Patsy's, and it's a sunny day, I'm in a good mood, and I'm determined to eat well at lunch. As I get into the parking lot of Patsy's, I make sure I remind myself to eat well, because I know that I'll feel better afterward, as well as look better in the long run. I imagine myself walking up the stairs, sitting down with my friends and then the bread plate comes—but I ate an apple before I sat down, and had a bottle for water so I wasn't starving . . . Leaving

Patsy's, having eaten a healthy meal and not going off my life program . . . let's see . . . I'm in my car on the way back to the office, I'm driving, and instead of feeling bloated, guilty, and disappointed in myself, I feel accomplished, like I'm on my way to living a healthy life, losing weight, looking better . . . I even imagine myself fitting into a size-8 dress . . .

You see, the idea is to go through in your mind, imagine the entire thing, this way you will be prepared—mentally rehearsed.

I also ask the waitperson to bring out a plate of raw or cooked vegetables so I can nosh on that while we wait to order.

You must go through and really understand the experience with *conscious* thought. When you set goals, it's important to think through the motions and visualize what it takes to get through the rough times—it helps to think through the details and it gives you time to plan in advance. Don't fly blind—give yourself the advantage—you deserve it.

8. **Write down some of the images.**
   Which ones were the strongest? Which ones made you feel the best?

9. **Focus on the visualization of your primary goal frequently.**
   Give it positive energy with strong affirmations and feelings that the goal is real and reachable.

10. **Avoid negative thoughts.**

If negative or self-sabotaging thoughts come into your mind, replace them with the feelings and images you created and the increasing feelings of success and competence as you take each step.

OK, now take out a notepad. Start by picking your goal, sitting in a comfortable environment, and begin by allowing yourself to dream about it. Then start the process of writing it all down.

Still Having Trouble?

If you struggle to visualize where you want to go, you may want to consider seeking out the advice of a mentor or coach who can take an objective view of you, your situation, and your capabilities. Ask this person how she might see you in the future if you were stretched to the limits of your capabilities. It should be someone who has a lot of faith in you. There's a good chance that she will come up with ideas that never occurred to you, and that these ideas will, in turn, trigger some ideas of your own.

Knowing what you want is important, but it is just a part of the battle. Your thoughts and actions must be achievement oriented for you to reach your goals. You greatly enhance your chances for achievement by being proactive, setting goals, thinking positively, and effectively visualizing the end result.

Developing a Goal Planning Program

After understanding the detailed components of setting, creating, and planning goals, and once you have a firm grasp of visualization to prepare you for the hard work and obstacles that are inherent to goal planning, you need to break down the goal-planning process into some easy-to-follow steps:

Set a Primary Goal and Then Break It Down

Goal planning entails forming a strategy or plan of attack that includes the detailed steps that will take you there, or what psychologists call "sub-goals." Sub-goals are short-term goals or milestones needed to reach the much larger overall goal. Once you set an overall or primary goal, it should not remain at the forefront of your mind at all times. This would be overwhelming and even distracting from the business at hand. Your overall or primary goal, should be used for motivation, to keep you on track and focused on the "big picture."

Imagine if your goal were to get a Ph.D. Once you begin on that path and make your decision, you need to focus next on the *sub-goals.* Sub-goals need to be planned and thought through. In getting a Ph.D. you would need to focus on applying to graduate school, finding an advisor, choosing a thesis topic, and so on. Although getting your Ph.D. is your overall primary goal, each morning you get out of bed, you need to pay attention to your strategy and details, and be prepared for obstacles and changes in course that will occur along your path.

Another example: You've decided to write a science-fiction novel. But while you are in the process of doing so, you have numerous sub-goals: deciding on a theme, writing an outline, developing the characters, writing and rewriting chapters, fixing little plot problems, and if you are a first-time writer, finding an agent to sell it. If you think only of finishing the book, which is the larger goal, and don't carefully pay attention to the sub-goals, your chances of achieving your primary goals will be at risk.

Perhaps the best example of this is what alcoholics and other addicts do in order to stay sober. While the overarching desire is to, say, quit drinking, it inspires them to attend their first AA meeting; AA philosophy encourages them to "take it one day at a time." First, drinkers must stay alcohol-free, not just sober, for one day, then another day, then another. Many AA members say achieving these mini-goals is essential to their recovery and much less daunting than swearing to themselves that they will quit drinking forever.

You may be tempted to set more than one goal within each of the categories outlined below, but I would advise you to stick with one goal at a time (per category)—as long as you make it a sound, quality goal (see the details earlier in this chapter under "*What Makes a Good Goal?*"). Setting more than one goal can dilute your efforts, and provide you with an excuse for failing to reach either goal.

What is a quality goal?

One that's important to you, something that has been nagging at you for a long time, or something that will significantly improve the quality of your life. Career, personal fitness, and relationship goals are all worth pursuing. If you have a problem such as an addiction to drugs or alcohol, there's no question that you need to tackle that problem before you can realistically set any other personal goals. But you don't have to wait until you accomplish one goal before you begin dreaming up and planning another. Goals can overlap. Don't rest on your laurels. Constant challenges keep you engaged in the miraculous process of living. The setting, planning for, and reaching of personal goals is a pattern worth repeating.

Breaking your goals down also includes preparing for the difficulties that aren't in your control. If you've decided to cut down on or eliminate sweets, you may face the possibility of being in a situation where sugar is the featured guest, as in a birthday party at home or at the office. Don't succumb either out of temptation, wishy-washiness, or the desire not to offend. In these instances, having a preplanned response can help you avoid such setbacks so just say, without apology, "No thanks!"

Goal Planning Example

The following is a detailed example to show you how goal planning is effectively broken down and reached. Review this closely, because I'll ask you to do your own goal planning right after this example.

Phase I: Goal Planning for Three Months to a Year

Primary Goal–Personal

The Goal:

To lose 20 pounds in the next six months and change my style of eating and exercise. I want to look great in a bathing suit, have more energy, and want people, including myself to find me attractive.

The Strategy, Specific Details, and Sub-goals:

1. *Exercise three times a week. Eat less fast food. Cook healthy meals at home.*

2. *When will you exercise? (e.g., two weekdays during lunch hour, one weekend morning.) Where? At the gym or elsewhere? What sort of exercise? (aerobics? walking? weight training?)*

3. *What will you eat? (Suggestion: Make a detailed list of delicious foods you can eat, a more positive tool than a list of forbidden foods.)*

Obstacles or Potential Setbacks I May Encounter in Pursuing These Goals:

1. *At family gatherings, I tend to overeat and throw my diet out the window.*

2. *Lunchtime at the office—once a week we go all go out to Patsy's and I eat the most fattening, calorie laden foods, and always have dessert.*

3. *I travel for my job and have difficulty maintaining good eating habits. I'm always eating on the run—in the airport, in the hotel, or in my car at a drive-thru fast-food restaurant.*

4. *My biggest problem is late-night snacking. Right after dinner I'm ready to sit in front of the TV and eat an entire new meal.*

"Plan B" — Ways to Overcome These Obstacles or
Potential Setbacks:

1. *Prior to family gatherings, I will decide to bring my own food or ask the host to prepare something special that is not high in calories.*

2. *Before our weekly lunch at Patsy's, I will make sure to call the restaurant and have them prepare a few low calorie dishes. I will make sure the waiter knows in advance. I will also use the visualization techniques outlined in* Breaking the Pattern *to mentally rehearse these weekly lunches.*

3. *When traveling on airlines, I will make sure to order a low-calorie special meal, or if unavailable, I will prepare a low-calorie meal for myself. I will make a focused effort not to eat in airports or in my car by thinking ahead and preparing foods in advance, or making sure there is low-calorie food where I'm going. I will make this a priority.*

4. *Again, I'm going to prepare for late-night cravings by preparing in advance. I will cut up vegetables, and other low-calorie snacks. I will also try to make sure I have my primary visualization goal in mind and use it to keep me focused. I will also*

take a walk or do some other activities during the most prob-lematic times.

Excuses I Might Use to Pull Me from My Goals:

1. *I only live once—why am I wasting my time trying to lose weight?*

2. *I'm genetically made this way.*

3. *I've tried to lose weight before and couldn't do it.*

Excuse Busters:

1. *I have only one chance at a good life. If I get sick because I'm overweight—it means I'm not doing my best to make my one time great.*

2. *Yes, I may be genetically inclined to be overweight, but I realize that I can control my eating, break my patterns, and learn new ones to make up for my genetics.*

3. *Trying and failing is not a strong reason not to try again. I know that losing 20 pounds can be done.*

Short-Term Rewards:

1. *Feel healthier in general.*

2. *Have more energy and not feel sluggish.*

3. *Decreased guilt due to overeating.*

Long-Term Rewards:

1. *Fit into a great-looking bathing suit.*

2. *Reduce my chances of getting one or more of the seven serious diseases related to being overweight.*

3. *Be happier and more self-aware.*

4. *Increase self-confidence.*

This type of detailed plan of attack will relieve anxiety and prepare you to tackle any challenges that come your way. Remember: Life is constantly surprising you and will likely come up with new obstacles to throw into your path. Don't set goals with a false sense of optimism that everything will go smoothly the first time. You may grow disappointed and frustrated that you'll be tempted to discard the goal as unreachable. In a college graduation speech, Governor James Martin of North Carolina said: "Instead of a false sense of optimism, I think it's better to visualize being calm in the face of adversity." In other words, *anticipate reality.* Make room for mistakes in your goal planning. Always be ready to readjust and keep on your path to your dreams. Be flexible. Revise if necessary.

Most of us spend time pondering goals that are immediately reachable. To get in touch with and make use of your inner visionary, be aware of all three of these time frames. In each time frame, you'll have career and creative aspirations, as well as personal ambitions, which can include goals for your relationships, fitness, personal growth, hobbies, and travel. Below are some charts that can help map out where you are and where you want to be three months to a year from now (Phase I), where you want to be in two to five years from now (Phase II), and what you want to have accomplished in 10 to 20 years (Phase III).

All three Phases are important. With each Phase, there's a career and work section that deals with your aspirations in business and in creative side to your life. The second section focuses on your personal life; it deals with all aspects, including but not limited to, your interpersonal relationships, family, and friends. It also includes all aspects of personal growth, health, fitness, hobbies, travel, and such. Of course, your goals will always change and vary, but what you write in these charts can be used as a guideline. The Phases and the sections are merely here to provide you with a starting point; they're not set in stone. Remember that although your goals will always change and vary, they hold enormous value to you as guidelines for the future. You should be as detailed as possible in filling out these sheets. Take your time filling in these sheets. Don't do them all in one sitting.

Phase I looks at the "near/near," covering about three months to a year from now.

Phase II looks at the "near/far," which projects two-to-five years from now.

Phase III looks at the "far/far," or where you want to be in the next 10 to 20 years and beyond.

I'll break down goals into different categories:

▶ Career and Work
▶ Relationships and Family
▶ Health and Wellness
▶ Religion and Spirituality
▶ Personal Improvement, Hobbies, Learning and Education

EXERCISE 1
Phase I: Goal Planning for Three Months to a Year

Using the following breakdowns as a guide, you can begin your goal planning and excuse busting for your *Career and Work Goals* for Phase I: *Three Months to a Year from Today*. After your *Career and Work Goals*, apply the same breakdowns to clarify your goals in terms of Phase I for your *Personal Life*. Although it might be a bit overwhelming, try including a separate Phase I for each of the following under *Personal Life:* relationships and family, religion and spirituality, health and wellness, personal improvement, hobbies, learning and education. You should try to create one primary goal for each area, or you can simply start with the two most important areas.

My Primary Goal—Career and Work:

The Goal:

    1.

    2.

    3.

The Strategy, Specific Details, and Sub-goals:

    1.

    2.

    3.

Obstacles or Potential Setbacks I May Encounter in Pursuing These Goals:

    1.

    2.

    3.

"Plan B"—Ways to Overcome These Obstacles or Potential Setbacks:

    1.

    2.

    3.

Excuses I Might Use to Pull Me from My Goals:

    1.

    2.

    3.

Excuse Busters:

    1.

    2.

    3.

Short-Term Rewards:

    1.

    2.

    3.

Long-Term Rewards:

    1.

    2.

    3.

My Primary Goal—Personal:

The Goal:

    1.

    2.

    3.

The Strategy, Specific Details, and Sub-goals:

    1.

    2.

    3.

Obstacles or Potential Setbacks I May Encounter in Pursuing These Goals:

    1.

    2.

    3.

"Plan B"—Ways to Overcome These Obstacles or Potential Setbacks:

    1.

    2.

    3.

Excuses I Might Use to Pull Me from My Goals:

    1.

    2.

    3.

Excuse Busters:

    1.

    2.

    3.

Short-Term Rewards:

    1.

    2.

    3.

Long-Term Rewards:

    1.

    2.

    3.

EXERCISE 1

Phase II: Goal Planning for Two-to-Five Years

Using the following breakdowns as a guide, you can begin your goal planning and excuse busting for your *Career and Work Goals* for Phase II: *Two to Five Years From Now.* After your *Career and Work Goals,* apply the same breakdowns to clarify your goals in terms of Phase II for your *Personal Life.* Although it might be a bit overwhelming, try including a separate Phase II for each of the following under *Personal Life: relationships and family, religion and spirituality, health and wellness, personal improvement, hobbies, learning and education.* You should try to create one primary goal for each area, or you can start with the two most important areas.

My Primary Goal—Career and Work:

The Goal:

    1.

    2.

    3.

The Strategy, Specific Details, and Sub-goals:

    1.

    2.

    3.

Obstacles or Potential Setbacks I May Encounter in
Pursuing These Goals:

    1.

    2.

    3.

"Plan B"—Ways to Overcome These Obstacles or Potential Setbacks:

    1.

    2.

    3.

Excuses I Might Use to Pull Me from My Goals:

    1.

    2.

    3.

Excuse Busters:

    1.

    2.

    3.

Short-Term Rewards:

    1.

    2.

    3.

Long-Term Rewards:

    1.

    2.

    3.

My Primary Goal—Personal:

The Goal:

    1.

    2.

    3.

The Strategy, Specific Details, and Sub-goals:

    1.

    2.

    3.

Obstacles or Potential Setbacks I May Encounter in Pursuing These Goals:

    1.

    2.

    3.

"Plan B"—Ways to Overcome These Obstacles or Potential Setbacks:

    1.

    2.

    3.

Excuses I Might Use to Pull Me from My Goals:

    1.

    2.

    3.

Excuse Busters:

    1.

    2.

    3.

Short-Term Rewards:

    1.

    2.

    3.

Long-Term Rewards:

    1.

    2.

    3.

Phase III: Goals for 10 to 20 Years

Using the following breakdowns as a guide, you can begin your goal planning and excuse busting for your *Career and Work Goals* for Phase III: *10 to 20 Years From Now.* After your *Career and Work Goals,* apply the same breakdowns to clarify your goals in terms of Phase III for your *Personal Life.* Although it might be a bit overwhelming, try including a separate Phase III for each of the following under *Personal Life: relationships and family, religion and spirituality, health and wellness, personal improvement, hobbies, learning and education.* You should try to create one primary goal for each area, or you can simply start with the two most important areas.

My Primary Goal: Career and Work:

The Goal:

    1.

    2.

    3.

The Strategy, Specific Details, and Sub-goals:

    1.

    2.

    3.

Obstacles or Potential Setbacks I May Encounter in Pursuing These Goals:

    1.

    2.

    3.

"Plan B"—Ways to Overcome These Obstacles or Potential Setbacks:

    1.

    2.

    3.

Excuses I Might Use to Pull Me from My Goals:

    1.

    2.

    3.

Excuse Busters:

    1.

    2.

    3.

Short-Term Rewards:

    1.

    2.

    3.

Long-Term Rewards:

    1.

    2.

    3.

My Primary Goal—Personal:

The Goal:

1.

2.

3.

The Strategy, Specific Details, and Sub-goals:

1.

2.

3.

Obstacles or Potential Setbacks I May Encounter in Pursuing These Goals:

1.

2.

3.

"Plan B"—Ways to Overcome These Obstacles or Potential Setbacks:

1.

2.

3.

Excuses I Might Use to Pull Me from My Goals:

1.

2.

3.

Excuse Busters:

    1.

    2.

    3.

Short-Term Rewards:

    1.

    2.

    3.

Long-Term Rewards:

    1.

    2.

    3.

Once you have made your goal lists, try to determine which ones are the most essential to you. On a scale of one to ten, rate your level of commitment to each one. Use visualization and mentally rehearse how you plan to go about each of the steps required. Think of how it will feel, look, sound, smell. Keep the end goal in mind. How do you feel about each of your goals? Are some more important than others? Focus on the ones that are most essential.

Your goal sheets serve as little road maps you have created for your life. While you may want to focus on one goal at a time, you should keep your overall goal sheets on hand, and periodically consult them. You may have to redraw the map from time to time, but at least you have some idea of where you want to go.

The next Principle, *Achievement,* will take you through other key steps to get your goals on the mark.

Summing Up

▸ Practicing visualization helps you to break out of a rut, or break-through an obstacle. It can raise your expectations about your life and what you'd like to achieve, help you define your goals, then motivate you to reach them.

▸ Visualization is *daydreaming with a purpose*. You're exploring who you are, and getting to know your aspirations and desires. Daydreaming without a purpose is not so bad either and can provide you with information about yourself.

▸ Visualization is essential because it infuses you with a sense of self-confidence, and makes you feel that your goals are both real and reachable. It gives you energy and desire and helps maintain motivation.

▸ There are ten basic steps for visualization:
  1. Get comfortable;
  2. Close your eyes and dream;
  3. Concentrate on something you would like to achieve or simply let your mind wander;
  4. Now, bring your thoughts in and be specific about your goals;
  5. Think about what it would feel like to achieve your goal—dream consciously;
  6. Visualize the details;
  7. Get further into the details, break every component down including the sub-goals;
  8. Write down the strongest visual images;
  9. Return to your visualizations frequently, give them positive energy with strong affirmations and feelings that the goal is real and reachable; and

10. If you have negative or self-sabotaging thoughts, replace them with the positive ones created in this exercise.

▸ Visualization is essential to help you get comfortable with the notion of yourself as a person who can accomplish your goals. Before figuring out how you're going to get there, you need to know in detail where you want to be, and visualization makes that happen.

PATTERNS
FAILURE
RESPONSIBILITY
GOALS
ACHIEVEMENT

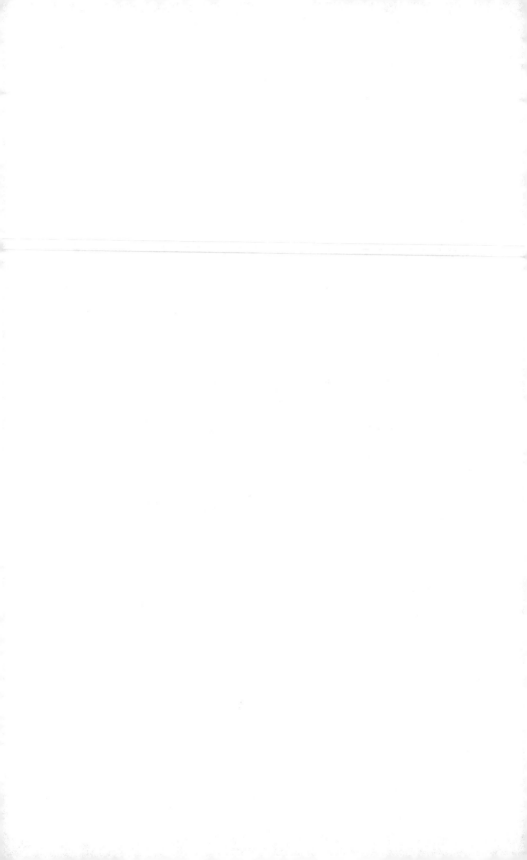

CHAPTER SEVEN

Making Change Happen and Transforming Your Life

*It is not the critic who counts, not the man who points out
how the strong man stumbles or where the doer of deeds
could have done better. The credit belongs to the man
who is actually in the arena, whose face is marred
by dust and sweat and blood, who strives valiantly,
who errs and comes up short again and again
because there is no effort without error and shortcomings,
who knows the great devotion, who spends himself in a worthy cause,
who at best knows in the end the high achievement of triumph and who,
at worst, if he fails while daring greatly, knows his place
shall never be with those timid and cold souls who knew neither victory nor defeat.*
—Theodore Roosevelt

Originally, I named this last Principle in the book *Success*, and I even thought about calling it *Transformation and Achievement*. After thinking it through, I realized the objective is not success, but *the tactics and strategies required to create movement in a positive direction*. To reach your goals, achieve, or succeed, you not only need to recognize patterns, understand failure, and take responsibility—but you also need effective methods of change to help you on your mission toward *Breaking the Pattern*.

Achievement vs. Success and What Each One Really Means

"Success" is a glitzy word. It conjures up visions of bucket loads of money, the esteem of others, and a life of prosperity. Attractive as they may seem, surprisingly, these are *not* universal goals. More importantly, you should achieve something meaningful in life, reach your goals, and actualize your potential.

Since I believe that it's richer and ultimately more fulfilling, I am more interested in talking about *achievement* rather than success. One definition of achievement, courtesy of *Webster's*, is "to get by effort." Another definition is "to bring to a successful end." As these definitions imply, achievement and success are intertwined. However, *they are not interchangeable.* Often, success, along with wealth and admiration, flows naturally from achievement.

This is all well and good, but how do you decide what you want to achieve and where it can take you? Some of you are stuck at the starting gate. Or, you have not even decided yet what race you want to run. In other words, you don't know what you're passionate about, and have no idea what goals you want to pursue.

The following Principle will help you delve deeply into the various techniques that people of high achievement use to set, plan, and reach their goals. If you're drawing a blank, the following information and exercises will help you tap into your imagination and release ideas and dreams as you work to develop a more fulfilling life. I'll walk you through a few mind-expanding exercises using techniques that have been proven to work, including *affirmation, self-talk, paradigm shifting, proactive behavior,* and other methods for transformation and achievement.

Remember: Breaking the mold and shaking things up a bit is what it's all about. Real life is not necessarily about getting things right, but instead about taking risks, experimenting, making mistakes, and even failing. Change creates things and makes things happen. That's what achievement is—reaching your goals. And that's the real payoff!

Some people are lucky enough to be clear about what they want to accomplish in life from a very early age. I'm sure you knew people like that in high school. They seemed to know just where they were going and had their path all mapped out. But many of you struggled with an abundance of indecision, more or less falling into jobs, relationships, and friendships without much deliberation. You've largely let life happen to you.

If you've just begun to plan and create goals, and still feel confused about how to achieve them, it helps to start off with an exploratory process. This involves a few steps. Your exploration needs to be *external* and *internal.* It's *external* in that you need *to be open to and aware of the opportunities around you, and internal,* in that you need *to be keenly aware of your own values.* Next, do not let others determine your idea of achievement, and when and if you should achieve. Lastly, you need to know yourself and your history well enough to recognize and *remember those experiences in life that have been optimal, ones during which you have felt "in the flow."* Learn these three approaches so that you consistently reach your goals.

Let's examine them one at a time beginning with opportunity:

Opportunity Ready

The key to breaking any pattern is the desire to change. When you're ready to change, you'll begin to open up to new circumstances. Being open and ready to change are critical components to propel you toward your goals. There is a saying, "When the student is ready, the master will appear," which means if you're ready for change and transformation, the material you need to make them happen will come to you. Opportunities surround you. If you make it a point to be aware of and open to the world you're familiar with, you might find long-overlooked answers to problems that have plagued you. If you are close-minded—unwilling to explore new ideas and review your current situation—it's unlikely you'll even see an opportunity, even if it's right smack in front of you. The failure to see these solutions has sometimes been called *resource myopia*. That is, you don't see what's under your nose because you're so close to it. There are many examples of this around you—like when the boy next door turns out to be the love of your life. The world of business offers many examples of people who recognized a great enterprising idea just by being attentive to their everyday world and making connections between experiences.

Howard Schulz, the founder and CEO of Starbucks, is an example of a leader who noticed and embraced opportunity around him. Originally from Brooklyn, Schulz was working for Hammarplast, a houseware corporation in New York. He began to notice an intriguing phenomenon: a small retailer in Seattle was placing unusually large orders for a certain type of drip coffeemaker.

As he recounts in his book, *Pour Your Heart Into It*, Schulz decided to take a trip out to Seattle to investigate. What he found was a small but thriving business, called Starbucks, run by coffee connoisseurs who roasted and sold whole-bean coffee for people to brew at home. He was enthralled, both by Seattle and by Starbucks, so he took a pay-cut and started working for them.

When he began, he expanded their coffee-roasting business. Then, on a trip to Italy, while walking the streets of Milan, Schulz had an epiphany. He noticed the prevalence of small espresso bars and how they acted as meeting places and cultural centers of neighborhoods. He also noted that people were willing to pay for high-quality coffee drinks. "This is so powerful, I thought. This is the link . . . What we had to do was unlock the mystery and romance of coffee, firsthand, in coffee bars. The Italians understood the personal relationship people have to coffee, the social aspect. I couldn't believe Starbucks was in the coffee business, yet was overlooking such a central element of it. It was like an epiphany. It was so immediate and physical that I was shaking . . . If we could recreate in America the authentic Italian coffee-bar culture, it might resonate with Americans the way it did with me. Starbucks could be a great experience, not just a great retail store."

Of course, not everyone saw the opportunity as Schulz did. The owners of Starbucks resisted the idea of selling coffee by the cup on a permanent basis. So Schulz decided to open his own coffee bar. He approached 217 investors and 214 of them said they wouldn't invest in Starbucks. Americans did not want to sit around and drink dark, expensive coffee, they told him. They just want to grab a cup of the ordinary stuff and go. But Schulz was indefatigable. "I never once believed, not ever, that my plan was not going to work," he says. Later he admitted, "There's a fine line between self-doubt and self-confidence, and it's even possible to feel both simultaneously."

With the support of a few dedicated investors and employees, he opened his first coffee bar, called "Il Giornale," in downtown Seattle, and introduced Americans to the "latte." Before long, his business grew so successful that he was able to buy out Starbucks coffee roasters, and the name. But he was just beginning. He envisioned Starbucks all across America, not just in urban centers, but also in neighborhoods everywhere. "Instead of a small dream, I dreamed big," he recounts, "After all, who wants a dream that's near-fetched?"

Being Ready and Knowing It

As you've already learned, I've struggled with weight loss and fitness for twenty years. The last time around, about six years ago, I lost 50 pounds and kept it off. I know I've achieved my goal through extensive research, hard work, *and* by following my own advice. But most of all, *I was ready and open to change.*

Understanding this concept is critical.

You need to open yourself up in order to free your mind and expose yourself to new influences. Think of your mind as a bowl or a jar with a limited capacity, once it's full, that's it—you can't fit in anything else. When you free yourself up, there will be room for new additions.

Helen Hunt, the Emmy and Oscar award-winning actress, acknowledged, ". . . the only time I've moved forward in my career is when I had the courage to say 'no' to things that were safe or that I'd done before, in order to create a space for something new to enter." It's true, and obvious, that you can't do everything and anything that you want to because there's only so much time in the day. Thus, you need to break old negative patterns and replace them with new, positive patterns. This mind-set will allow you to be ready to accept change, movement, and transformation. *Remember: In order to seize opportunity, you have to be open to it and aware that it exists.*

Another area in my personal life in which this concept became clear is my relationship with women. I found myself dating a woman who was absolutely wrong for me. She was consistently inconsiderate, always late, completely irresponsible, and had no interest in personal growth, but it didn't matter. The truth was, I wasn't ready to be in a long-term relationship that could lead to marriage, and in part, I stayed in the situation to keep myself in a "safe" place—one in which I knew I would never have to make a commitment. I kept myself in a comfortable place, and as a result, I had no room to meet another person—I was "full." After years of dating this woman, we finally split up and it opened me up to meet my life partner.

I recently heard a story of a man who had been divorced for about five years—he was deeply hurt by the break up and fearful of falling in love again. He immediately met a woman who he began dating, but he made it clear to her that he wouldn't marry her, ever. Dating this woman protected him from having to fall in love with someone and the risk of being hurt again. After realizing he was ready to commit, he separated from this woman and, now, for the first time, he can conceive of meeting someone and feeling love again. He needed to be ready and open for change to occur, and his first step was getting out of a relationship that didn't provide for commitment.

Allowing and preparing yourself to open up and be ready for change is a critical component of breaking patterns. Remember: *Opportunity favors the prepared mind.*

EXERCISE 1
Opening Up to Opportunity

Many people come up with great ideas or solutions to problems by changing their physical environment. When I travel, the change in routine frees up my mind and I do my most creative thinking. List three methods you will use to create free flowing thoughts so you're open and ready to embrace opportunity and change. What will you do differently to break out of the mold? Some examples include simply sitting in a room for 30 minutes with no distractions, taking a long walk or hike, or even a quick day trip. List your ideas below.

Know Who You Are, Where You Stand, and Your Value Knowledge

Values are not just morals; they are all the things we hold dear. All of us have a hierarchy of values. How do you discover yours? For starters, try to be attentive and aware of your responses to events and situations. As you go about your daily routine, ask yourself to define what is most important to you. A nicely designed room? A relationship with a friend or lover? The quality of the food you eat, or even coffee you drink? Where and how you get to your job each morning? What TV shows you choose to watch? Your political views? When you watch a movie, what do you find yourself responding to? The acting? The music? The story? The costumes? Who are you down to the core?

So, what is *value knowledge?* It's becoming aware and being conscious of who you are and what you want. Every experience offers a window into yourself and reveals what you value most. Pay attention to these. You need to look at who you are in order to determine what you want. And why is this so important? By paying close attention to the people in your life, what you do each day, and how you do it, you open yourself up to developing the self-awareness that's necessary to break patterns, and ultimately live a happier and healthier life.

When I discuss success and achievement in this book, it relates to specific values and goals that *you* set for yourself. There are no judgments here, except the ones that you place on yourself. If you value staying home and sitting on the coach and eating bags of chips, I simply say: that is *your choice* and recognize that you have made that choice because that's what you want to do. Awareness creates choice, and knowing your values is part of awareness. So the bottom line is: If you're conscious of what you want and why you want it, you'll have a better chance of moving in that direction.

Remember: This book doesn't say: *"You can get whatever you want whenever you want it."* It only serves as a guide that tells you: *"You have control and are responsible for the directions that your life takes.. You can make a difference. You will not always reach your goals, but there is a better chance if you follow the steps mapped out in this book."*

EXERCISE 2
Learning Your Values

Take your time and ask yourself the following questions—remember to be honest:

1. If you did not have to make a living, what would you do with your time?

2. Is there a way to turn your hobby into a living?

3. What did you enjoy doing most as a child, before you had grown-up responsibilities?

4. What do you like to do with your "free" time?

The second important part of knowing your values is this:

Don't Let Others Determine Your Future

For some people, terms like "success" and "achievement" immediately conjure up images of the rich, powerful, and famous. Try to let go of those associations.

Be wary of any undermining cultural blocks or barriers to change that may have been instilled in you from a very young age. Among them could be a lack of playfulness, lack of curiosity, or other internal boundaries that hold you back. Many of you have been taught that it's wrong to look at things differently from the rest of society and that you must conform. These prescriptions can make you lose confidence in yourself so that you view reality and opportunities only in terms of the categories or structure that others set forth. *Don't let others dull your sensibilities.*

Dream the great dream, imagine the impossible, and fantasize (just like you did when you were a child). The idea is to free your thoughts, free yourself of ordinary routines, and allow yourself the opportunity to think "outside the box."

Give yourself the time to review. Take a look at the routines in your life and make sure that you're following the path you want to follow. Remember that behavior often becomes automatic—you develop a life momentum from which your patterns emerge. Examples include: 1) taking people or situations too much for granted; 2) you no longer truly observe what's going on in your life; 3) you assume you've seen it all, or can predict what will happen. Think of it this way: When you reread something you've written for the third or fourth time, you're so familiar with the content that you just skim over it and don't catch the mistakes.

Instead, you need to keep a fresh perspective of yourself and get feedback from trusted sources. The idea is to develop these skills so you can monitor your own behavior, keep tabs on yourself, and keep yourself on track.

Many therapists and psychologists call this idea of watching your own behavior an *observing ego*. This concept can be likened to having an out-of-body experience. Use the "observing ego" to gain as much objectivity as possible. By taking a step back from your everyday interactions with others, you become aware of the role you play in shaping your behavior and circumstances. The "observing ego" should help you monitor your goals and aspirations, and keep you operating on the path that you've set for yourself.

It's also important to make sure that you *are* taking risks without worrying whether or not you're making other people happy by conforming to *their* wishes and goals. Recognize that you need to be willing to "fail" and learn from your mistakes in order to experience the life *you* want. Finally, you should always take into account that entering something new is not always comfortable. Just like a new pair of shoes, it takes time to get that "worn-in feeling."

Remember, this doesn't mean that you throw everything that might stand for security and stability out the window and leave your spouse, quit your job, and move to some far away land. Living a balanced, examined life that's true to your own values is important—so keep things in perspective. Take steps that you feel comfortable with—dance to your beat, not to someone else's.

EXERCISE 3
Playing It Safe

List four current situations, relationships, or circumstances in which you think that you take the "safe route." Perhaps your daily routine has gotten the best of you or you're just terrified of failing. Be specific and don't just make a list: note the reasons why and how you are being held back. While doing this Exercise you should remember everything discussed in the previous chapter on *Responsibility*—and remain aware of the fact that you are solely responsible for how your life unfolds.

Ideally, you should do this Exercise by going to a place you have never been before. Take a drive or get on a bus, even if it means staying in the same town—just somewhere different. Spend the day in this different environment if you can. Negative aspects come with almost every decision you make but to move forward, you must assume a certain amount of risk. Remember not to berate yourself while doing the Exercise (hint: Review Chapter 3 on *Failure*).

Here's an example of how to complete the Exercise: You can say to yourself, "I've been living in the same city and apartment in the northeast for the last 20 years, even though my dream is to live in a warm, rural environment on lots of land. I feel safe, I know the area, and my job is here. I could ask for a transfer, but what if they fire me, what if I leave my house and my job, and I don't like the new area?"

Now list 4 "safe/comfort" areas of your own that hold you back.

1.
2.
3.
4.

Okay, now for each one of these situations think of a way to take more risk, open up opportunity, and free yourself to move forward. Don't be afraid of this Exercise. Yes, for many it's scary to even think about ways to increase risk, let alone writing them down on paper. Remember: Just because you write it down doesn't mean you have to carry it out. For example, (taking the next step from wanting to relocate) you may write: "I'll explore houses on the Internet that are in the vicinity where I'd like to live. Maybe I'll even call a few brokers. I'll also review some of the companies I could work for in those areas, maybe even redo my résumé." So, in this part of the Exercise, you don't have to actually move to the new house, just talk about the steps toward assuming a little more risk.

1.
2.
3.
4.

In the movie *Any Given Sunday*, Al Pacino plays a pro football coach. In the locker room, he delivers a speech to his players about winning *inch by inch*. He says that you find that life is a game of inches because the margin for error in either game, football or life, is so small. "One half-step too late or too early and you don't quite make it. The inches we need are everywhere around us, they're in every break of the game, every minute, every second . . . we claw with our fingernails for that inch 'cause when you add up all those inches, that is what makes the difference between winning and losing.'"

Okay, so it's a little much, but I think you get the point. The idea is to take baby steps (if you need to) and achieve your goals by moving inch by inch. In another movie, *What About Bob,* a comedy staring Bill Murray and Richard Dreyfus, one of the many themes focuses on taking small steps to break through negative patterns. Dreyfus' character, a psychiatrist, writes a book called *Baby Steps,* exactly on this topic. You don't have to take giant steps or pray for the miracle of chance to "score," to reach your desired results.

Get Into The Flow—Finding Your Positive Patterns

At some time in your life, you may have had the feeling of being completely in the moment, completely focused on what you were doing, and immune to all distractions. What were you doing at the time? Were you painting? Cooking? Playing a sport? Some describe this feeling as being "in the zone." Others say, "I was feeling it." Some call it being "in the flow." A psychologist once dubbed these *optimal experiences,* tremendously productive and satisfying events in which the *act of doing* follows with extreme ease—*it just feels right.* Wouldn't it be nice to always have that sensation?

Michael Ray, a Stanford Business School professor, explains: "It's like the experience you have when you make a perfect shot in a tennis match or say just the right thing in a meeting or make just the right move in a relationship. That experience tells you that there's something really great inside of you—that you're somebody who can hit that perfect shot, and that you can probably hit it all the time." The idea is that these moments, your "Aha!" moments, are proof positive that you do have what it takes.

Think back to when you were "in the flow" and try to replicate what you did to get there. Chances are you were passionate about whatever activity it was that allowed you to tap into this "flow" experience. When you're working your way through a goal/task that you're not as passionate about, it's tougher to reach that optimal place—it just means putting in more effort.

Always look for clues to your real passions. People who are very successful and who achieve a great deal need to be passionate, as well as disciplined about their pursuits. Without passion, the work will become pure drudgery.

During the Sydney Summer Olympic Games, *The Wall Street Journal* wrote a story about Dr. Simons, a Californian who works as a sports psychologist for the Australian Olympic team. Dr. Simons practices "one of the least understood" roles in sports. In a world where performance is measured to the millimeter and by the microsecond, the contribution of a sports psychologist can't be quantified, or easily detected. "Most people think we use some kind of magic, that we're gurus or ultra-motivators," says Dr. Simons, known to his athletes as "The Psych." In fact, the message he drills into athletes is simple and straightforward. He tells them to "become the eye in the hurricane"—calm, focused, and undistracted.

"Positive thinking is great, but there's a cold hard reality to sports that you can't escape," he said. "You can 'visualize' beating Marion Jones all you want, but the best psychologist in the world can't help you win if your body isn't up to it."

It is very difficult for individuals to get to the (mental) place that will drive them to perform to the best of their ability. "Very few people in their entire working lives experience one moment as intense and pressured as this," Simons said. The trick, according to him, is helping athletes to be their best in the race of their lives, against the world's best, before a crowd of 110,000, with cameras beaming the action everywhere in the world.

You may not need to work toward such championship moments on a daily basis, but you should work toward opening up your mind for opportunity and achievement. The main objective of a sports psychologist is to help athletes find "that clear white spot inside where they perform best." This is exactly what you need to find in your life. To do this, Simons urges athletes to study themselves and "pattern" the state of mind in which they've excelled. He says they're often surprised to realize they've done best when relaxed, almost not caring, rather than being all "keyed up." In this respect, a good part of achieving, succeeding, and moving forward relies on "The Three C's": calm, cool, and collected.

Personal Energy

To accomplish your goals, you also need to sustain *personal energy*. While personal energy cannot be quantified, you know what it feels like when you're drained of it. If you're lucky, you also know what it feels like to be full of energy and ready to conquer the world. What you do to your body, how much you sleep, and what you eat and drink significantly impacts your energy level. But emotional events and how you react to them also affect you physically. Unless you're very good at changing gears, stressful, unrewarding days exhaust your energy, causing you to be distracted from other commitments and projects.

But when all systems are harmonious, the human body/psyche becomes a remarkable producer of energy. People who are enthusiastic about what they're doing can work long hours, sometimes with less sleep, and still wake up restored and raring to go. When, you're "in the zone," "in the flow," or having an "optimal experience," energy is not even an issue. Why can't you feel like this all the time? Can you set up your life so that you feel it more often?

Frustrating and repetitive activities deplete energy. The result is exhaustion, detachment, boredom, depression, and in the extreme, paranoia. When confronted with these feelings, you lose the ability to think straight. You start putting more energy into finding excuses to avoid work than into work itself. Your efforts become less and less productive.

Receiving encouragement from others and feeling good about your efforts is energizing, just as negative feelings sap you of energy. You can't expect to feel positive about every aspect of your life at all times. Use self-knowledge as your first line of defense against energy-draining, negative responses to life experiences.

Here are some questions to ask yourself and Exercises to improve your understanding of your own personal energy:

EXERCISE 4

Energy to Burn

---

1. What are your high and low points of energy during the day? When are you most productive and clear thinking? If possible, can you schedule important events for your best time of day, and make full use of that time? Are there activities you can schedule during your lower energy times that might be less taxing, but still productive, and even potentially re-energizing?

2. What aspects of your life frustrate and drain you of energy? Do they tend to be associated with a certain time of day? With one particular person? How do they arise and work themselves out? Do your actions and reactions to the situations contribute to your frustrations? Is there one small aspect of your own behavior or attitude that you could change that might change the whole dynamic?

3. As an experiment, try shifting your attitude about a certain task

or job or person from negative to positive for a day, or if you can't muster that, for just a few hours. Emphasize the positive aspects about a person or task that you have previously seen as a problem. Decide not to let it get to you. Smile. See if, at the end of the day, you feel less drained than usual.

Changing your outlook from negative to positive is not easy. *It's crucial to remember that you, alone, are responsible for your responses, attitude, and reactions to things.* You create your own emotional climate. Do not cede that responsibility or power to anyone else.

There are various tricks for replenishing personal energy. Affirmations, visualization, and meditation are effective because they calm the mind and body, relieve stress, improve concentration, increase energy, and allow you to listen to your intuition and stay true to your personal goals. These cost nothing, and even a short session of any of them can be helpful. You need only to decide to give yourself a moment alone to perform them. Ultimately, they work better than any over-the-counter energy boosts (caffeine, sugar, ginseng, etc.) that many people fall back on. These stimulants provide you with a spurt of energy, only to send you crashing down a few hours later.

Motivation

Motivation is important to understand in the scheme of things. *What motivates you to do what you do?* Is it money, status, approval, keeping up with others, a drive to win, doing the best you can do, always learning and improving? If you figure out what motivates you, you've taken a giant step toward replacing your negative patterns, and establishing new, more positive ones to reach your goals.

A person's motivation results from many factors, including education, culture, ambition, self-confidence, rearing, and much more. You must review the roots of your motivation, specifically in regard to your negative patterns. Not only do you have to identify and recognize negative patterns, you need to explore the motivations that support those behaviors.

EXERCISE 5

Why Are You Still Doing It?

Review five negative patterns that you discovered in the chapter on *Pattern Recognition* (page 37) and note the underlying motivation that supports them. In other words, ask yourself why you're choosing to continue the negative patterns that currently exist in your life.

EXAMPLE

Negative pattern: *Smoking*

Result: *Poor Health.*

My motivation: *Smoking makes me feel better, so I choose to smoke.*

1. Negative pattern:

   Result:

   My Motivation:

2. Negative pattern:

   Result:

   My Motivation:

3. Negative pattern:

   Result:

   My Motivation:

4. Negative pattern:

   Result:

   My Motivation:

5. Negative pattern:

   Result:

   My Motivation:

Summing Up

- ▸ Seize opportunities. Solutions need not come from far away to be important, effective, or obtainable. Remember that in order to seize an opportunity, you have to be aware that one exists.

- ▸ Open yourself up and free your mind to allow for new influences; they can make all the difference.

- ▸ Understand your value knowledge. This means you're aware of who you are and what you want. Every experience offers a window into yourself and reveals what you value most.

- ▸ Be wary of any undermining cultural blocks or barriers to change that may have been instilled in you at a very young age. Among them are a lack of playfulness, lack of curiosity, or other internal boundaries that might hold you back—cut them loose.

- ▸ Look to your optimum moments for inspiration. Think back to when you were "in the flow" and try to replicate what you did to get there. Chances are you were passionate about whatever activity it was that allowed you to achieve this "in the flow" experience.

- ▸ Know what motivates you to do what you do. Is it money, status, approval, keeping up with others, a drive to win, doing the best you can do, always learning and improving? Once you figure out what motivates you, you take a giant step toward breaking existing negative patterns and establishing new, more positive ones.

CHAPTER • EIGHT

Tactics and Strategies for Changing Your Life

A lot of what we ascribe to luck is not luck at all.
It's seizing the day and accepting responsibility for your future.
It's seeing what other people don't see, and pursuing the vision,
no matter who tells you not to. . . . While bad luck, it's true,
may come out of the blue, good luck, it seems, comes to those who plan for it.
—Howard Schulz, founder and CEO of Starbucks

Responsibility is when you stop saying, "Why me?" and start saying
"What next?" The minute you take responsibility, you become more creative.
—Julia Cameron

As we've discussed, achievement is not just luck—there are proven methods and specific techniques to break patterns, reach your goals, and improve the overall quality of your life. Part II of *Achievement,* focuses on these methods: affirmation and self-talk, expectancy theory and the placebo effect, paradigm shifting, and proactive behavior.

Affirmation and Self-Talk

An affirmation is a strong positive statement that assumes something desirable *is, in fact, true.* The act of using words and "talking to yourself about yourself" makes affirmation more real than just visualizing it regardless of how detailed the vision might be.

Whether you're aware of it or not, most people's lives are accompanied by a stream of internal commentary. An example would be constantly telling yourself "I can't lose weight—it's just too difficult" or "I'll never get promoted. I'm stuck in this dead-end job forever."

Would you ever get on an airplane after you overheard the pilot say, "I don't think I can make it all the way to Florida. I just know I'm going to crash, I'm so scared . . ." No, of course not. Aren't you the pilot of your own life? You're the one in charge; do you really want to be the one convincing yourself that you will not succeed? Granted, there are times when it's natural to feel insecure about your undertakings—but don't be your own worst enemy. Take a risk and believe in yourself.

As one researcher points out, "The formula is simple: Knowledge plus congruent beliefs equals action." If you're down on yourself, you may be constantly berating yourself with negative talk. As an alternative, affirmations perform three very useful functions:

▸ Make you aware of your own thoughts.
▸ Replace negative thoughts with positive ones.
▸ Reinforce positive thoughts and feelings.

This helps you to identify existing thoughts and replace those that don't support achievement-directed goals with those that do. When practiced and repeated over time, affirmations can alter your mental climate and empower you to make changes in your life. Most of you are familiar with the children's book, *The Little Engine That Could*, in which a humanized "choo-choo" train is able to surmount challenges that seem impossible by chanting over and over "I think I can, I think I can." This is a parable about the power of affirmations. And, as automotive pioneer Henry Ford said in a similar vein, "If you think you can't, you're right."

Affirmations are a particularly focused version of self-talk. Both are used a lot in the world of sports. Jim Johnson, a sports psychologist for professional sports teams, teaches athletes to replace negative self-talk with positive statements. If you make a mistake, don't scold yourself, he suggests. "Acknowledge your frustration, let it go, and focus on the next play." He instructs the players to constantly tell themselves reassuring thoughts like, "I am a major league baseball player," or "I'm going to throw nine innings today." Like most sports psychologists, Johnson believes that baseball is only 25 percent physical. "The difference between Triple A ball players and big leaguers is mental," he told *U.S. News and World Report*.

You too, can reap the benefits of reassuring self-talk; it will help you deal with your frustrations and keep you on track. The key to using affirmations effectively is to overcome what I have previously called "the corniness factor." You may be reminded of Al Franken's goofy and hilarious character ("Saturday Night Live"), Stuart Smalley, and his mantra: "I'm good enough; I'm smart enough; and gosh darn it, people like me."

You may laugh at yourself when you start to use affirmations. It's okay to laugh. Affirmations do sound funny at first. Eventually, when you're comfortable with the idea of yourself as someone who can achieve your dreams, you'll become more comfortable with the strategies to live them.

EXERCISE 1
Begin Thinking of Affirmations

I recommend writing your affirmations down in the present tense, and repeating them to yourself either as a kind of meditation and/or whenever you are experiencing a situation in your life that normally upsets you, causes you or damages your self-esteem. For the person who experiences problems on the job, such an affirmation, would be something like: "I am a competent person who is capable of succeeding at this task." For an overweight person who struggles with a poor body image, the affirmation might be something like: "I am a beautiful person and I deserve to look the way I want to look." The repetition of such positive statements will eventually lead to a change in the way you view yourself and your own capabilities. Gradually, the mind responds affirmatively and you begin to experience your intended results.

What Happens When Things Change?

It's very important to remember change can feel awkward, and just because it feels strange doesn't mean it's wrong (and just because it's comfortable doesn't mean it's right). Many times your "comfort zone" is comfortable simply because you've been there for such a long time. This is how a pattern continues. Anytime you start something new, it feels different than usual. Have you ever moved your residence? What were those feelings like? Probably pretty strange. It probably took a while to get used to, but once you felt comfortable, it was like you had always been there. It's similar to buying a new pair of shoes—at first they're stiff, many times they even hurt, but over time, the leather molds to your feet, and eventually they become your old favorites.

The process of self-reflection and self-assessment is critical to living a conscious life. Be prepared for change, open yourself up and embrace opportunity.

EXERCISE 2

The Experience of Change

Write down three life-changing experiences:

1.

2.

3.

What were the results of these changes? Review each one of these. Did you eventually become accustomed to the change?

1.

2.

3.

Expect It, and It Could Happen

Throughout the history of the self-improvement industry in America, one simple yet challenging idea has prevailed: If you believe it in your mind first, it will happen. Yet until recently, there hasn't been much scientific evidence suggesting that thoughts can translate into biological action. Medical researchers investigating the phenomenon of *placebos* on the healing process have taken the first steps toward understanding the pathways from thought to action.

A placebo has been described as "typically a sham treatment that a doctor doles out merely to please or placate anxious or persistent patients. It looks like a drug but has no pharmacological properties of its own." Placebos, like sugar pills, have been used in the scientific process to determine the real effectiveness of a drug. By giving a specified number of unknowing test subjects a placebo (and the same number of unknowing test subjects the test drug), it's possible to determine the real effect of a drug compared to the imagined effect. What controls the experiment is that *all* test subjects have been told what the drug being tested should do.

There are many stories throughout medical history that attest to placebos being as powerful as the actual drugs they were tested against—sometimes even more powerful. A famous example is that of "Mr. Wright," a California resident in the '50s, who was diagnosed with cancer and was given only days to live. He had tumors the size of oranges but had heard that scientists had discovered a horse serum, called Krebiozen, that was effective against cancer. He repeatedly asked his doctor to treat him with it, and his doctor finally agreed. Within days, the doctor reported, "The tumors melted like snowballs on a hot stove." Mr. Wright was "the picture of health" for a few months before he read a report that the serum was, in fact, proven to be worthless against cancer. Mr. Wright died two days later.

Undoubtedly, these sorts of stories fuel popular myth, yet there has always been a question as to how much healing can be attributed to placebos. Recent research has changed the old notion of placebos as "quack" medicine. Using techniques of brain imagery, scientists continue to learn that the placebo effect is even more powerful than anyone had once thought. This investigation suggests that a host of biological mechanisms can turn a thought, belief, or desire into an agent of change in cells, tissues, and organs. From it they have started to deduce that much of human perception does not rely on information flowing into the brain from the outside world but rather on what the brain expects to happen next based on previous experiences.

This is a remarkable statement, not only for the future of medical treatment, but also for the future of self-management. It begins to substantiate what psychologists and self-help gurus have long believed: Mind can succeed over matter. Positive thoughts can produce change for the emotional mind and biological body.

Dr. Irving Kirsch, a psychiatrist at the University of Connecticut who carried out a recent review of placebo-controlled studies on antidepressant drugs, found that placebos worked about as well as their genuine counterparts. "If you expect to get better, you will," said Dr. Kirsch. Clearly, there is still skepticism in the medical community (much of it undoubtedly fueled by pharmaceutical companies that would stand to lose billions of dollars). Nonetheless, a variety of studies have shown the effectiveness of placebos for treating everything from asthma, allergies, and joint repair, to hair growth and pain management. For example, doctors in Texas conducted a study on arthroscopic knee surgery in which patients with sore knees were given one of three operations: scraping the joint, washing out the joint, or nothing at all. Those who received nothing at all reported the same amount of relief from pain and swelling as those who underwent the real operations.

In his book, *The Healing Power of Faith*, Harold Koenig, M.D., a professor at Duke University Medical Center, found that people with strong faith in a supreme being—an intimate and intentional God—have an advantage in healing because of this belief. In fact, one study showed that nonreligious patients with heart disease were three times more likely to die following surgery than their religious counterparts. It's important to keep in mind Koening's distinction between "simply the forces of faith," versus faith put into action, which reaps the highest rewards for individuals.

Why do placebos work?

The answer to that question may lie in the area of cognitive neuropsychology called *expectancy theory*, which explores "what the brain believes about the immediate future." It seems that much of what the brain believes is based on what it has experienced previously. Like Pavlov's dog that salivated at the sound of a bell—the classic conditioning theory—people associate healing with the trappings of medicine. That is, for most people, the medical treatments a person receives throughout life produce an expectancy that things such as a doctor's white coat, a needle's prick, or a pill, will bring relief from pain or will effect a cure.

Scientists have recently begun to realize how closely the brain is linked to the immune system and the hormone-producing endocrine system. They are still trying to determine exactly how these systems operate when a placebo is introduced. A placebo may simply reduce stress, or there may be special molecules that carry out placebo responses. Somehow, scientists continue to find that expectancies are embedded in the brain's neurochemistry. As Howard Fields, a neuroscientist at University of California at San Francisco, says, "We are misled by the dualism or the idea that mind and body are separate."

An example of how expectancy works in ordinary life is as follows: Have you ever seen someone at a distance walking toward you and you say to yourself, "Isn't that . . . ?" You see a familiar face, but when you get closer, you realize it's a stranger. How does that happen? Some features like hair color, or face shape, led you to expect the person to be someone you know. Your brain then quickly filled in the other distinctive features (the eyes, ears, etc.) and transformed the person into someone you know. Because you thought you knew that person, you had a certain response. If you had had a bad experience with that person in the past, you might become anxious, nervous, and begin to sweat. Your body creates a response to something that you believe to be true.

In fact, many psychologists claim that individuals can have a "learned helplessness," a situation in which an individual seems preordained to fail. Therefore, if you're expected to do poorly, there is a greater likelihood you will do poorly. I remember being tested as an elementary school student, and the results showed that I was weak in certain subjects. Well, I ended up being weak in those subjects, until one teacher took a keen interest in my ability. This teacher hadn't seen the specific test results, and expected me to be successful, and eventually, my grades increased.

There have been studies in which teachers have been told certain children were of exceptional intelligence, and others had slight learning disabilities. In reality, the children were all of equal intelligence levels. In independent tests, the students who were considered exceptional performed substantially better than those who were considered less intelligent.

The exciting future of expectancy theory holds many possibilities for improving your life. In fact, you can use the notion of expectancy to help you accomplish your goals. If you want something, it may or may not happen. But if you expect it to happen, and you visualize it clearly, you can greatly increase the chances of it happening. You can trick the brain into thinking it is inevitable by using affirmations, self-talk, and other techniques. If you think it, believe it, cause others to believe it—you can effect change.

Self-Efficacy and Expectancy Theory

Albert Bandura, a Stanford University psychologist, said, "People's beliefs about their own abilities have a profound effect on those abilities. Ability is not a fixed property; there is a huge variability in how you perform. People who have a sense of self-efficacy bounce back from failures; they approach things in terms of how to handle them rather than worrying what can go wrong."

To be both personally responsible and proactive, you must believe in what Bandura calls *self-efficacy, a situation-specific self-confidence* or belief in yourself. His theory describes how people's expectations lead to behavior. In essence, Bandura said, there are two kinds of people: those who believe they personally have the ability to act in a way that produces a desired outcome, and those who believe more generally that *their* actions are not directly related to desired outcomes. The difference is self-efficacy.

Let's take the example of someone who's trying to manage his weight. The person must believe that he alone can modify eating and exercise patterns to lose weight, not just accept the general belief that changing these patterns can lead to weight loss. Therefore, he needs a deep belief in his own ability to change, rather than holding onto a vague sense that somewhere out there in the world, people can change their lives.

Nothing builds confidence in your self like successful past experience. By surmounting obstacles and reaching goals, you reinforce belief in your self-efficacy. People who have quit smoking, controlled their weight, learned to manage pain, rehabilitated themselves after a serious illness or injury, or even stuck to an exercise regime, also get the added bonus of a deeper level of confidence in themselves that will likely serve them well in other aspects of their lives. But which is the chicken and which is the egg? In some cases, you have no idea what you are capable of until you are put to a real test. Though some are lucky enough to have a background and/or parents who have fortified their confidence and hope, self-efficacy is not something that people are born with. It is something that comes over time with experience. And ideally it is *learned and cultivated.*

One way to begin is with small steps. Take one small thing in your life that you'd like to change and carry it through. Rather than a complete change in all of your eating habits, eliminate one "toxin" from your diet, such as sugary soda. Maybe fast food. But really make it happen. Or, start taking a 10-minute walk at lunch everyday, and really stick to it. If you can succeed in changing in one small way, your confidence and pride, sense of possibility, and self-efficacy will all begin to expand.

Paradigm Shifting—Changing Negative Thoughts

Many years ago, I first heard the term "paradigm shifting" in the book, *Seven Habits of Highly Effective People* by Stephen Covey. With paradigm shifting, *your thoughts create your feelings.* It is further defined as your thoughts creating the choices you make. What a revelation, I thought. The concept is pretty simple to understand, but very difficult to master. *The bottom line is: You're responsible for your thoughts and feelings, and therefore, have the ability to change them.*

I'm not saying that you can't feel bad, or be upset, or have any other negative emotion, just that you're more in control of your thoughts and feelings than you might think.

Paradigm shifting is an important principle; in fact, in Stephen Covey's book, he lists it as one of the seven key habits. What does this mean for you and me? Basically, it means you can change the way you view things by going ahead and simply changing them. Wow, that concept is way out there! But to bring the discussion back down to earth a bit, all it really means is that situations can be viewed many different ways. What appears to be absolute is anything but.

In fact, a recent article in a business journal talked about trying to teach a similar principle to a group of ten executives. Researchers placed 10 men in a sand garden. The garden contained several huge boulders but they were buried so that only a small fraction of each boulder showed above the gleaming, manicured white sand. All of the executives were asked about the "rocks" in the sand. The executives assumed the rocks were small and could be easily removed; not considering the possibility that parts of the rocks might be hidden below. The executives didn't think much of the "small rocks." Once they realized the rocks were actually huge boulders, their perception and strategy shifted. Bear with me while I use a cliché to illustrate my point here: "Things are not always as they appear."

In an interview in *Fast Company*, Jeffrey Christian, CEO of Christian & Timbers, really drove home the point of creating your own opportunities and shifting paradigms:

"I spend about 40 percent of my time on the road, so I've reached the point where I expect to run into travel hang ups in one form or another, especially during the holidays. But when I walk into an airport, I have a completely different attitude from that of the disgruntled masses waiting for their flights and fretting about missed connections. That's because I count on the downtime to chat on the phone with friends and relatives."

Remember: The point here is not to completely disregard negative thoughts and situations. Only discount these thoughts and feelings once you have evaluated them and learned from them.

Changing Your Thoughts and Feelings

List three irritating/annoying situations you have encountered at work, and three with your family (or simply at home with a neighbor or friend). Then fill in where you might have thought differently, more positively, if you knew a particular fact or just simply had more information about the circumstances.

EXAMPLE

The incident: *"I prepared an elaborate anniversary dinner. My husband was late and I couldn't reach him by cell phone . . . I was worried and angry. The later it got, the angrier I got. I was ready to scream.*

Additional Information: *When my husband walked in and told me he was delayed because he helped save someone's life in a traffic accident.*

How your thoughts and feelings changed: *Well, when I found that out, I wasn't angry anymore. I was proud that he helped save someone and completely disregarded the fact that he was late . . ."*

Now, think about three irritating/annoying incidents *at work*:

   1. The incident:

      a. Additional information:

      b. How your thoughts and feelings changed:

2. The incident:

    a. Additional information:

    b. How your thoughts and feelings changed:

3. The incident:

    a. Additional information:

    b. How your thoughts and feelings changed:

Now, think about three irritating/annoying incidents *with your family or in a significant relationship.*

1. The incident:

    a. Additional information:

    b. How your thoughts and feelings changed:

2. The incident:

    a. Additional information:

    b. How your thoughts and feelings changed:

3. The incident:

    a. Additional information:

    b. How your thoughts and feelings changed:

Balance

What is balance? This subject could be a book on its own. Balance is defined in the dictionary as "stability produced by even distribution of weight on each side of the vertical axis: mental and emotional steadiness." It is being able to live a harmonious life—not too far to the right or to the left, but still enjoying the extreme highs life offers. Balance also means something else: To achieve anything you must realize you can't achieve everything. You want to excel at your job, be the world's greatest mother or father or lover, conquer the world, and climb Mount Everest. Many of you are pulled in various directions. You can't do it all, and you can wear yourself out trying. So how can you operate at your fullest capacity, right up to that limit, without burning out and fading away?

I believe the key is in finding your own individual balance, which is *different for everyone.* Some people can work 12 hours a day and stay focused and excited about their work. Entrepreneur and television host Martha Stewart always talks about how she works 20 hours a day and sleeps only 4, and it works for her. But others would curse every minute of a 12 or 20-hour workday. Some can get by with 4 hours of sleep, others need 14 hours. Some simply do not want to spend that much of their life either working or sleeping. They pursue other interests, hobbies or avocations; or they spend time with their families.

These equations can change at different times in our lives. The essential thing is to either derive some contentment from the course you are on, or change it. Keep asking yourself: "Am I still learning, growing, pursuing, and fulfilling my goals and passions?"

Achievement and workaholism are not one and the same. Simply working long hours and moving through life at breakneck speed does not indicate personal growth. Once, during his tenure at Chrysler, Lee Iacocca overheard one of his senior vice presidents bragging that he hadn't taken a vacation in 2 years. His reward? Iacocca fired him on the spot. In a magazine interview he said that someone who hadn't taken a vacation in 2 years had something "seriously wrong with him."

The old adage is right: You must work at what you can control and not worry about the things that are beyond your control. It's no simple matter to strike that balance. Too much acceptance can turn you into a passive and eventually regretful victim. Too great a need to control can bring about perfectionism and demanding behavior to the point of sabotaging your chances for achievement and happiness.

EXERCISE 4
Spy on Yourself

An effective way of assessing the balance in your life is to keep a daily log for 2 weeks. Record all of your activities, their duration, who is there with you, the results. There should not be any time gaps. Try to make this an accurate and precise account of how you spend your days and to what end.

After 2 weeks, look it over to get a better sense of how you spend your time, and whether it matches your goals and aspirations, and if it is enjoyable. Pay careful attention to how you feel about your log. Ask yourself these questions using your "observing ego":

1. If this person whose life you see on the page were not you, how would you describe him or her?

2. Does this person on the page seem to spend all of his or her time working? Playing?

3. Is work/play time fulfilling?

4. Is this person moving toward attaining his/her goals?

5. Does there seem to be something missing from this person's life?

6. Would you choose to be friends with this person? Why or why not?

7. Would you choose to work with this person? Why or why not?

Being Proactive

Only an infant believes that his needs should be entirely met by other people. After all, he's a genuinely helpless being, unable to do much more than cry and hope that someone hears him. Once you're about 2 years old, you become actively interested in controlling your environment and in doing things for yourself. All of your early childhood development is geared toward independence and self-determination—from learning how to speak to learning how to walk, you are programmed to want to control your future. Yet, as adults, you might give up on that idea, and place control, actively or passively, in other people's hands.

The ability to rebound after setbacks and failures depends on your willingness to take responsibility for them—and this is no different for the business world. According to one study by the Center for Creative Leadership, business executives who experienced setbacks were much more likely to spring back quickly when they took responsibility for them. Those who became defensive about failure, or tried to conceal it or blame others for it, had a much longer, difficult road to travel.

Successful managers admit when they've miscalculated and they try to correct their errors, learning from them along the way. There are several reasons for this. Remember the old bromide that states: those who do not learn from their own mistakes are doomed to repeat them. Or the other: The search for excuses and/or others to blame is time-consuming and futile. You may think you're sparing yourself unpleasantness and pain by handling failure this way, but you are only prolonging it.

So then why is taking responsibility such a hard thing to do? I believe it's because you still see it as a negative thing—a weight and a burden—rather than an opportunity for self-empowerment. You may also tend to think of responsibility as something to do after the fact, after things have already gone wrong. But the most effective way of taking responsibility is before the fact—proactively.

To be proactive is to act in anticipation of a future problem. You can often anticipate future problems from past experiences. It's much easier to educate individuals on fire prevention, then to put out a burning building.

When you take responsibility you're not merely reacting to life's many circumstances; you're also anticipating problems and taking steps to avoid them. You're plotting your own course and not leaving the planning to others.

You may tend to think of taking responsibility as something you do after things have already gone wrong. This is often just a way of setting yourself up for failure, of not being fully invested in your own success, and awarding yourself with the convenience of having someone to blame. But where does this get you? Granted it *may* spare you some sorrow in the short-term. It was Sophocles who said: "The keenest sorrow is to recognize ourselves as the sole cause of our adversities."

Thus, proactivity.

Being proactive is the opposite of being reactive. It is acting before the fact rather than after. Reactive people are often strongly affected by externals. If the weather is good, they feel good. If not, attitude and performance suffer. Proactive people, however, carry their own weather with them. Rain or shine, they are in good form because they write the script. According to Siddhartha, the founder of Buddhism, the Buddha said if you want a smooth journey in life, all the roads should be covered in leather. But since that is impossible, Buddha said you should wear leather shoes. By this he meant, deal with problems before they arise.

Being proactive also means knowing your strengths and acting on them. Being proactive means taking time to plan out where you want to go. Proactive people take bold, imaginative steps to create and seize opportunities, rather than waiting for opportunity to come knocking on their doors.

Anticipation—An Example of Proactive Behavior

The discussion on *Patterns* touched upon *ego defense mechanisms,* and how repression, denial, rationalization, and intellectualization are ways we cope, however ineffectively, with anxiety. The good news is that there are productive and mature ways of shielding yourself from anxiety—ways that do not block necessary truths from your consciousness or prevent you from assuming responsibility for your personal actions. The most important and healthiest tool for dealing with anxiety is *anticipation.* It is also something that can be implemented easily, and will become a pattern with a little practice. Anticipation eases you into situations, sees you through deep feelings, and helps you take responsibility.

Anticipation is realistic planning for discomfort and/or anxiety. For example, a family with a terminally ill grandmother will undergo some anticipatory mourning so the inevitable loss does not come as too great of a shock and overwhelm the family's ability to cope. Another example of the effects of anticipation is delayed gratification. When you put off watching a movie to study, or pass on that piece of chocolate cake in order to stay trim, you are anticipating rewards down the road.

Lisa's case is a good example.

Lisa's long-time boyfriend, Dan, recently broke up with her—she was devastated. Unfortunately, Dan still lived on the same block in New York City as she did. As a result, Lisa was terrified of leaving her house on the chance that she might run into him. Her fear of such an encounter drove her to humiliating behavior such as ducking behind bushes on her way to work. Lisa knew she was being ridiculous, but she did not feel up to dealing with the shame and embarrassment of seeing Dan again. What if he were with another woman?

I offered her one solution in jest: move to another neighborhood.

"But this is New York City," she protested. "You know how hard it is to find a good apartment in this city. I'm not giving mine up for anybody."

I thought that spark of defiance was a good sign. It showed she was taking some responsibility for caring for herself. I asked her to tell me the worst possible scenario she could imagine if she ran into Dan on the street. She answered, "That he would be with some supermodel and just blow right by me without a word."

Then I asked her. "Now, would that be the worst thing that has ever happened to you?"

She agreed that it would not, but she was still unsure. "I just know that I would be so shocked to see him and I would blabber like a fool."

I suggested that it was the element of surprise of running into him on the street that was scaring her. So, to prepare for that, why not plan out how she would react? Then, if the situation arose, she would know what to do. By *mentally rehearsing* the meeting—and *anticipating the situation*—she could reduce the anxiety she felt. Lisa decided it would be better not to tell Dan all she wanted to say right there on the street. It would be better to sincerely ask him to call her later. Through anticipation and mental rehearsal, her anxiety lifted.

I believe the following 4 stories showcase proactivity at its best. The first is about movie director, Steven Spielberg whose career could easily be summed up with the phrase, good things come to *those who will **not** wait.*

Steven Spielberg started in Hollywood at the ripe old age of 17 and he's now a legend in the movie-making genre! One day, the teenage Spielberg, then an amateur maker of 8mm films, took a tour of Universal Studios. On the tour, he met Chuck Silvers, head of the studio's editorial department. "He talked to me for about an hour," Spielberg later recounted. "He said he'd like to see some of my little films, and gave me a pass to get on the lot the following day. I showed him about 4 of my 8mm films. He was very impressed." A few days later, Spielberg borrowed his father's briefcase, to give himself an air of professionalism, and walked into the studio. He did not ask permission. He did not wait until he graduated from college to set up an appointment. He just walked through the gate. In his own words:

"There was nothing in the briefcase but a sandwich and two candy bars. So, everyday that summer, I went in my suit and hung out with directors and writers and editors and dubbers. I found an office that was not being used and became a squatter. I went to a camera store, bought some plastic name titles and put my name in the building directory: STEVEN SPIELBERG, Room 23C."

Listening to Spielberg talk about the gumption he had at 17 should inspire you to create such an opportunity for yourself, no matter what your age. Spielberg's audacity to walk into a studio and assume the role of a working director was true proactivity. Many of you might have taken such a daring risk when you were a teen-ager, but as you grew older, you accepted the dictum to follow the rules, and consequently lost faith in your ability to create amazing possibilities for yourself. If you achieve moderate success and security by following the rules, you can easily fall into the trap of depending solely on other people to create opportunities for you. Ultimately, this strategy leads to disappointment. Proactive people recognize their highest priorities and goals and take on all of the responsibility for reaching them.

Sumner Redstone is a *profile in determination* and courage in a different way than Spielberg. Redstone, the chairman of Viacom, survived a Boston hotel fire in 1979 by clinging to a third floor window with one severely burned hand. He maintained his composure, he later explained, by counting to 10 over and over. His legs were burned to the arteries and the tendons in one hand were destroyed, forcing doctors to amputate his little finger. The doctors never expected him to live through the 60 hours of surgery. He did. They told him he would never be able to walk again. He did. In fact, he exercises daily on a treadmill and plays tennis regularly, wearing a leather strap that enables him to grip a tennis racquet.

This refusal to accept the limitations imposed on him by a horrific accident exemplifies the outlook and approach that took Redstone from his family's drive-in theater business to being the CEO of one of the biggest media conglomerates in the world, Viacom, which owns Blockbuster Video, Paramount Communications, and cable networks like MTV, Showtime, Nickelodeon, and more.

Redstone always demonstrated a relentless will to thrive and a fair degree of entrepreneurial ingenuity. After serving as an intelligence officer in World War II, Redstone put himself through Harvard Law School by buying merchandise with GI discounts and selling them to local department stores for profit. Today, he considers his modest background—and the effort he expended to overcome it—one of his greatest assets.

He took over the family's Boston area drive-in theater business and turned it into National Amusements, a theater chain that operates more than 800 screens in a dozen states. He achieved this tremendous growth by taking personal, hands-on responsibility for every facet of the operation. One of his competitors, and his tennis partner to this day, Alan Friedberg of Loews Theaters, told *Time* magazine: "He'd call the head of a movie company over a single movie in a single town. Saturday or Sunday, he did not care. He'd do whatever he had to do legally to get the picture away from me."

Redstone was also a pioneer in the theater business, with an uncanny ability to spot trends early and a sophisticated talent for proactivity. In the '70s, he came up with the concept of multiple-screen theaters, copyrighting the Multiplex name. In the '80s, when he saw that cable TV and VCRs were hurting movie attendance, he engineered a takeover of Viacom, Inc., already one of the world's hottest TV properties. In the '90s, he bought Blockbuster Video and won the bidding war for Paramount, which went on to make such successful films as *Titanic.*

Those who observe Redstone in action have described him as relentless when it comes to getting what he wants. It helps that he also knows what he wants. Surprisingly, he does not care about leading an extravagant lifestyle. Despite the fact that *Forbes* magazine ranks him among the country's richest men, with a net worth of about $4.2 billion, he is known for living a humble and modest existence. For this man, possessions are not the point. Achievement is.

Betty Anne Waters is another example of someone who took action to change the course of her family's life. She watched helplessly in 1983 as her brother Kenny was convicted of first-degree murder—a crime she was convinced he didn't commit. Waters hired lawyer after lawyer to appeal the case but eventually the money ran out. She made a promise to her brother that she would prove him innocent of the charges, and she intended to keep that promise. She decided that she was going to get a law degree and appeal the case herself. The problem was that this single mother of two had only a General Equivalency Diploma, the equivalent of a high school diploma. Water's first order of business was to get her associate degree, and then a bachelor's degree in economics from Rhode Island College. While earning money as a waitress, she entered law school in 1995—12 years after her promise to her brother. While in her third year of law school, Waters did a research paper on the science of DNA testing, and realized its significance with regard to her brother's case.

After graduating from law school in 1998, and passing the Rhode Island and Massachusetts bar exams, Waters began her brother's appeal. She had a clerk at the courthouse in Cambridge locate a box of evidence from the trial so a DNA test could be done on the 19-year-old items with blood on them.

After 18 years in prison, Kenneth Waters was freed in March of 2001, thanks to his sister's proactive behavior.

Jack LaLanne has surely changed America's ideas about fitness. After a troubled childhood, Jack experienced a transformation in his teens. He dropped out of school, was underweight and pimply, and an extremely poor eater. Family history was not on his side. His father died young due to poor nutrition. At age 15, Jack attended a lecture on health, and vowed to change his life. Now considered the godfather of fitness, LaLanne invented the "jumping jack," among other achievements.

In peak condition, at the age of 49, LaLanne decided to set up a test: he wanted to prove it was possible to escape from Alcatraz by swimming to Fisherman's Wharf in San Francisco, but he did it handcuffed and shackled while towing a 1000-pound boat. At 70 years old, he repeated the feat, slightly modified—handcuffed, shackled, and battling currents, he towed 70 boats holding 70 people for a mile and a half across Long Beach Harbor. At 83 years old, he still works out 2 hours a day.

Despite what seems like a lifetime of devotion to physical fitness, LaLanne told *Esquire* magazine, "It starts up here. Right between the ears." He also confessed that he seldom feels like exercising. "Every day, I don't feel like working out. Shit, leave a hot bed and a hot woman and go into a cold gym at five in the morning. It's discipline. Pride and discipline. I work out first thing in the morning to get it the hell out of the way. Takes me two hours. An hour with the weights and an hour in the pool. At seven, my conscience is clear. I can look myself in the mirror and say, 'Jack, you've done it again.'"

While most of you might not match LaLanne's discipline, you can learn to take a more proactive role in your diet and exercise regimes.

Michael Dell is an example of proactivity because of his belief in *the importance of adaptability*. It's common in the business world for the founder of a company to lose control of it when it expands. From the McDonald brothers of hamburger fame, to Steven Jobs' first stint at Apple Computers, maverick entrepreneurs are often unable or unwilling to make the adjustment to being CEO of a much larger corporation. Not so with Michael Dell. The former whiz kid is still in charge of the computer company he started as an undergraduate at the University of Texas in 1984, and is the youngest person ever to head a Fortune 500 company.

Dell exhibited a proactive and entrepreneurial spirit early in life. At age 12, he made $2,000 by trading stamps through a mail-order catalogue. In high school, he turned his newspaper route into a serious money-making venture by targeting likely new subscribers. For example, he obtained the names and addresses of newlyweds at the local marriage bureau, and then sent them a personalized advertisement offering a special deal. With his $18,000 profit, he bought a BMW and shocked the car dealer by paying in cash.

At the University of Texas, Dell majored in biology, but computers fascinated him. At the time, retail stores sold standard personal computers at high mark-up prices and employed salespeople who knew little about the product. Dell thought of a better way—selling customized computers directly to consumers through telephone orders. He convinced retail outlets, such as ComputerLand, to sell him their surplus stock at cost. Dell assembled, customized, and souped-up PCs in his dorm room. Then he placed ads in computer magazines, courting purchasers who would recognize a good deal when they saw one.

The summer after his freshman year, he used his savings to incorporate as PC's Limited. He promised his parents he'd go back to school if his business did not immediately show signs of success. In its first year of operation, PC's Limited handled $6 million worth of sales, and the

University of Texas lost a student. In 1987, the company's name changed to Dell Computer Corporation, making Dell a household name. By 1988, sales had reached $159 million, by 1993, $2 billion, but by that time, the Wall Street favorite had stretched itself too thin.

The company had grown too fast without the necessary infrastructure and planning, and the stock was tanking. Dell recognized the problem, *took responsibility*, then took the unusual step of deliberately slowing the company's growth. By hiring a team of experienced industry executives to run the day-to-day business operations, he was free to focus on his strengths: developing technology and recognizing market trends. Although the price of Dell shares still fluctuates, the company remains a true success story.

Reaching "Aha!"

Everything you've done and all that has happened to you translates into an "experience." Most of you view your history through tinted glasses. Now that you've taken a good hard look at responsibility, you're ready to go back to the histories you wrote out in Chapter 2 (page 37). Try to see the patterns as they truly are. It takes years to develop them, and many are deeply ingrained. But it only takes an instant to make your mind up to make a change—the "Aha!" moment.

To recap, this is not the same as the trigger moment, which we discussed before. A trigger is an event that forces you to realize you want to make a significant change in your life. *The Aha! moment is when you see how that change will be made.* You see the light at the end of the tunnel, and the path toward reaching your dreams becomes clear.

For example, if you are dumped in a love relationship, you'll likely engage in a lot of self-reflection. You may decide that you never want to feel this bad again, that something has to change. That's a catalyst or a trigger. The Aha! moment comes when you realize how to do it, how you will change your negative patterns. You'll likely see your responsibility for the failed relationship, and enter into the next one with a better sense of yourself and, just as importantly, with a plan. Sometimes these moments visit you out of the blue, but you can help the process along.

Take Cheryl, a public relations executive, and mother of two, who has worked hard all of her life building her career and raising her family. At 42 years old, she found that she was repeating patterns in both major areas of her life—work and family. She was ending her second marriage, and completely dissatisfied with her position at the firm where she was working.

Cheryl's second marriage ended up being very similar to the first. Both husbands were very controlling, very successful, with "traditional values," and not very interested in fulfilling anyone's needs but their own. These were the same men she dated in college and in her premarital days.

As far as Cheryl's career, she took jobs because she thought they were sexy and fun, but they always ended up being boring, and very narrowly focused. She almost always complained about her boss, and about the company where she worked. "They do everything wrong, I'm surprised they can find their way to work in the morning . . ."

For Cheryl, applying the 5 Principles from *Breaking the Pattern* was a huge undertaking. In a terrible state, she had lost her job and was in the middle of a divorce. To make matters worse, she had gained almost 30 pounds as a result of all the stress and pressure. Cheryl's biggest obstacles were: Her reluctance to review her patterns by learning from her past mistakes and acknowledging responsibility for her situation.

It took about a year of struggle after her "triggers" converged before Cheryl began to notice substantial rewards from her process of change. As her first order of business, Cheryl evaluated her job; it seemed like the simplest place to start. She applied the 5 Principles, and used the Exercises. She was able to determine a common pattern in the companies that she worked. Most were small, and relatively disorganized. Cheryl seemed to be intimidated by large, organized companies. She felt she wouldn't be needed, and as a result, wouldn't last very long. She also believed that at a disorganized company it would be easier to look good, and if she made any mistakes they could be easily covered up.

Cheryl recognized her pattern, took responsibility, revitalized her level of confidence, and focused her energy on finding an appropriate company to work for.

Cheryl had the most trouble breaking her destructive patterns with men. It was difficult for her to see her mistakes, and even more so her responsibility, when it came to the men she had dated and married. She consistently argued that the men were all charming, not controlling, and very caring in the beginnings of the relationships. But "as soon as they felt secure—the flood gates opened. How could I be responsible for their behavior?"

It took a while before she could understand she wasn't responsible for "their" behavior, but for her own. She *chose* to stay in those relationships. Cheryl first had to identify her patterns for each situation. "It seems as if it's such a simple task, but it's not when you're in the thick of it. I always thought of myself as an aware, conscious person. When I started writing down and reviewing my history it all became much clearer. It didn't happen overnight, but over a period of time I started to see my patterns more clearly."

Understanding responsibility, and then putting it into practice, is a wonderfully liberating experience. Only then, you know that you have choices. As Cheryl said, "I thought I took too much responsibility for things that were going on in my life. I never would have dreamed it was the opposite."

In terms of her relationships, Cheryl did break her pattern and is currently dating someone who cares about her needs, and isn't controlling or demanding. As far as being overweight, Cheryl fully grasped the concepts of "free choice" and was able to recognize that she was choosing to be overweight. She effectively shed the extra weight by changing her lifestyle and paying closer attention to her reliance on overeating to soothe anxiety—it helped that she felt better about her job and personal life.

Summing Up

▸ Use affirmations, which are strong positive statements that assume something desirable is in fact true, to help you gain confidence. Talk to yourself about yourself only in positive terms.

▸ If you want something, it may or may not happen. But if you expect it to happen and if you visualize it clearly, you can greatly increase the chances of it happening. Train your mind into thinking that what you want is inevitable. You effect change.

▸ You're responsible for your thoughts and feelings, and therefore have the ability to change them. The miracle of taking action is that the way we view things can be changed by going ahead and simply changing them.

▸ Sustain your personal energy. Feeling good about your efforts energizes you, just as negative feelings sap you of energy. Use self-knowledge as your first line of defense against energy-draining, negative responses to life experiences.

▸ Stay in balance—live a harmonious life, not too far to the right or to the left, while still enjoying the extreme highs. Balance also means that to achieve anything, you must realize you can't achieve everything.

▸ Be proactive. Know your strengths and act on them. Proactive people take bold, imaginative steps, and create and seize opportunities, rather than waiting for opportunity to come knocking on their doors.

▸ Believe in and trust in your self-efficacy, a self-confidence or belief that you personally have the ability to act in a way that produces a desired outcome.

Investing in Your Success

After going through this book and having the courage to examine what you want as intensely as you have, I expect you're exhilarated if not completely exhausted. It takes a lot of work, understanding, desire, and plenty of discipline to get this far.

Although many of these concepts and exercises will make sense intellectually, it's challenging to put them into practice. Once you start making the Principles real by acting on them, interesting things will start to happen: You'll be able to clarify what matters to you and how to get it, and, you'll gain insight into how your friends, family, and business relationships work, and what they need to work better. You'll find yourself wanting to help others, and telling them what you've learned about breaking patterns—just like I'm sharing with you.

The exercises and information in this book have given you many of the tools you need to achieve your goals and succeed in your own way. How can you best put it all to use? You might be saying to yourself, "Hey, what's the payoff here? What am I going to get out of all the work I've done?" The best way you can answer this is to ask yourself: "Is what I'm currently doing working?" If so—don't change anything. But if not, well . . . what do you have to lose? If you want change, the power is within you.